HOLISTIC LIVING for WELLNESS

Your Guide to Spiritual Growth, Healthy Diet, and a Fitness Plan Even If Life Gets Busy

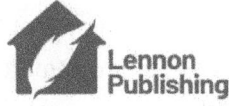

Lennon Publishing

Copyright © 2024 by Lennon Publishing

All rights reserved.

No portion of this book may be reproduced in any form without written permission from the publisher or author, except as permitted by U.S. copyright law.

This publication is designed to provide accurate and authoritative information in regard to the subject matter covered. It is sold with the understanding that neither the author nor the publisher is engaged in rendering legal, investment, accounting or other professional services. While the publisher and author have used their best efforts in preparing this book, they make no representations or warranties with respect to the accuracy or completeness of the contents of this book and specifically disclaim any implied warranties of merchantability or fitness for a particular purpose. No warranty may be created or extended by sales representatives or written sales materials. The advice and strategies contained herein may not be suitable for your situation. You should consult with a professional when appropriate. Neither the publisher nor the author shall be liable for any loss of profit or any other commercial damages, including but not limited to special, incidental, consequential, personal, or other damages.

Second Edition 2025

Contents

Note To The Reader   1

1. Foundations of Holistic Wellness   2
    Understanding Holistic Health: More Than Just the Body
    The Psychology of Self-Care: Why Your Mind Matters
    Emotional Wellness: Recognizing and Managing Emotions
    Integrating Mindfulness into Everyday Life
    The Science of Stress and its Holistic Counteractions
    Setting Realistic Wellness Goals That Resonate with Your Lifestyle
    Chapter 1 Wellness Plan: Introduction to Holistic Wellness

2. Nutrition for the Mind and Body   20
    Balanced Diets for Busy Professionals: Quick and Nutritious Choices
    Superfoods and Their Role in Mental Clarity
    Managing Dietary Needs Without Stress

The Impact of Hydration on Physical and Mental Performance
Planning Meals for Energy and Focus
Integrating Nutritional Strategies with Family Dining
Chapter 2 Wellness Plan: Nutrition for the Mind and Body

3. Physical Fitness in a Busy World   40
    Designing a Flexible Fitness Routine
    High-Intensity Interval Training (HIIT) for Time-Savers
    The Role of Walking: Underrated Exercises
    The Importance of Rest and Recovery
    Chapter 3 Wellness Plan: Physical Fitness in a Busy World

4. Mental, Emotional, and Spiritual Health Nourishment   62
    Practical Mindfulness Exercises for Anxiety
    Cognitive Behavioral Techniques Without the Jargon
    Building Resilience Against Daily Stressors
    Managing Social Anxiety Through Small Steps
    Enhancing Sleep Quality for Emotional Well-being
    Tech Tools That Aid Mental Wellness
    Art and Music Therapy: Creative Outlets for Stress Relief
    Chapter 4 Wellness Plan: Emotional and Mental Wellness

5. Spiritual Growth and Personal Faith   87
    Daily Practices for Spiritual Growth
    Meditation and Its Varieties: Finding What Fits
    The Role of Nature in Spiritual Wellness
    Creating a Personal Ritual for Spiritual Health
    Faith Across Cultures: Universal Wellness Lessons
    The Benefits of Spiritual Retreats in Everyday Settings
    Chapter 5 Wellness Plan: Spiritual Growth and Personal Faith

6. Sustainable Living and Wellness   108
    Eco-Friendly Choices That Enhance Personal Health
    Reducing Your Carbon Footprint with Smarter Food Choices
    Sustainable Fitness: Environmentally Conscious Exercise
    Household Toxins and Natural Alternatives
    The Wellness Benefits of Minimalism
    Community Gardening and Local Food Sources
    Chapter 6 Wellness Plan: Sustainable Living and Wellness

7. Social Wellness and Community Building   131
    Building Supportive Relationships
    Communicating Needs and Boundaries
    Volunteering: The Health Benefits of Giving Back
    Group Fitness and Social Bonds
    Online Communities for Holistic Health Support
    Wellness Workshops and Local Events

Chapter 7 Wellness Plan: Social Wellness and Community Building

8. Adapting Wellness Into Your Unique Lifestyle   153
   Tailoring Wellness Practices for Different Life Stages
   Overcoming the Guilt of Self-Care
   Integrating Wellness into the Workday
   The Role of Personal Development in Wellness
   Keeping Wellness Engaging and New
   Reviewing and Renewing Your Wellness Goals Annually
   Chapter 8 Wellness Plan: Adapting Wellness Into Your Unique Lifestyle

9. Bonus Chapter: Ask the Wellness Coach   177
10. Conclusion   184

References   188

Note To The Reader

Thank you for picking up the Second Edition of *Holistic Living for Wellness: Your Guide to Spiritual Growth, Healthy Diet, and a Fitness Plan Even If Life Gets Busy*

We've enriched every chapter with deeper spiritual reflections, refreshed meal templates and the brand-new bonus chapter "Ask the Wellness Coach," where real-world questions meet practical, down-to-earth answers. Your enthusiasm for the first edition's mindful practices inspired us to add even more tools for balance and inner calm.

Whether you're revisiting familiar ground or opening this guide for the very first time, you'll find playful prompts, nourishing rituals and candid Q&A designed to fit into the busiest of days. Dive in, explore at your own pace and let these pages support your body, mind and spirit—wherever life takes you.

Second Edition, 2025

Chapter 1

Foundations of Holistic Wellness

In the hustle of our daily routines, where deadlines, family obligations, and personal projects collide, the quest for health often becomes a footnote—a wishful note scribbled on the back pages of our minds. Yet, what if I told you that embracing a holistic approach to wellness could transform that footnote into the headline of your life's story, not just enhancing your longevity but enriching the quality of every moment? This chapter is dedicated to unfolding the layers of holistic wellness, a concept that integrates your physical, mental, emotional, and spiritual well-being, allowing you to thrive in a world that doesn't pause.

Understanding Holistic Health: More Than Just the Body

Holistic health is an invitation to explore wellness beyond the conventional scope. It's not merely about preventing or treating diseases; it's about nurturing a harmonious balance that enriches your life. This approach recognizes you as a complete entity, intertwining your physical, mental, emotional, and spiritual health. Take, for instance, how emerging research continues to reveal the profound connection between gut health and mental well-being. It's fascinating to discover that the simple act of nurturing your gut flora with a diet rich in fibers and probiotics can elevate your mood and cognitive function, illustrating a perfect example of how physical health impacts mental clarity.

Throughout history, holistic health practices have been a fundamental part of countless cultures worldwide. From the use of Ayurveda in India and traditional Chinese medicine in Asia to herbalism in indigenous cultures, these practices, though diverse in application, share a common principle: the belief in treating the individual as an interconnected whole rather than a series of parts. Over centuries, these ancient wisdoms have not only persisted but have also evolved, integrating seamlessly with modern medical practices to offer us a comprehensive view of health and wellness.

Contrasting sharply with conventional Western medicine, holistic health does not focus solely on symptoms but seeks to address the root causes of illness. Where traditional medicine might prescribe medication to relieve symptoms, a holistic approach considers the broader spectrum of an individual's lifestyle, environment, and emotional health. This might mean recommending changes to diet, exercise, social habits, and stress management as part of the treatment plan. It's a form of medicine that's as preventative as it is curative, emphasizing natural remedies and lifestyle changes over pharmaceutical solutions whenever possible.

Today, the acceptance of holistic health practices has seen a remarkable surge in modern healthcare settings. More physicians than ever before are prescribing integrative therapies like acupuncture, yoga, and meditation alongside conventional medical treatments. This shift reflects a growing recognition within the healthcare community of the benefits these ancient practices bring to modern medicine. For instance, hospitals incorporating stress-reduction programs based on mindfulness techniques have reported improvements in patient recovery rates and reductions in hospital stays.

As holistic health continues to weave its way into the fabric of modern medicine, it invites us to rethink our approach to health and wellness. It encourages us to consider not just the physical symptoms but the complex interplay of all aspects of our being. By doing so, it offers a more sustainable, empowering, and compassionate approach to healthcare, one that respects both the science of medicine and the art of healing.

The Psychology of Self-Care: Why Your Mind Matters

Understanding the role of mental health in overall well-being is pivotal. In our bustling daily lives, the mind often bears the brunt of our stress, juggling deadlines, relationships, and our aspirations. Research continually underscores the profound impact that stress has on physical health, ranging from weakened immune systems to increased risk of chronic diseases like hypertension and diabetes. The symbiotic relationship between mind and body is crucial for holistic wellness, emphasizing the importance of nurturing both mental and physical health for overall well-being. This intricate interplay highlights why mental health is not just a side note in the narrative of wellness but a central theme.

Self-care, often misconstrued as a luxury or indulgence, is a fundamental practice for mental health. Engaging in self-care activities like journaling offers a reflective pause from the daily grind, providing a space to process thoughts and emotions, leading to greater self-awareness and a reduced sense of overwhelm. Meditation, another cornerstone of self-care, allows for a mental breather, a moment to detach from the chaos of life and return with a calmer, more focused mind. Socializing, too, plays a critical role. It strengthens connections, provides emotional support, and often, a fresh perspective on personal challenges. The psychological benefits of these activities are profound—they not only enhance mood and energy levels but also fortify cognitive functions, making them essential tools in your wellness arsenal.

However, the path to regular self-care is often obstructed by psychological barriers. Guilt is a significant hurdle, with many perceiving self-care as selfish or unwarranted, especially when other responsibilities demand their attention. This guilt intensifies in a society that often glorifies relentless work and perpetual activity, neglecting the importance of rest and recovery. Overcoming these barriers begins with redefining self-care as a necessary practice that enhances our capacity to engage with life. By shifting the narrative to view self-care as an act of kindness to oneself, and by extension to those we interact with, it becomes easier to prioritize these practices without the accompanying guilt.

Cultivating resilience, essential for overcoming life's obstacles, is deeply intertwined with mindful self-care. It's about shaping a mindset that interprets obstacles as avenues for growth and perceives errors as essential steps in the learning journey. Such an outlook is fostered through mindfulness practices that emphasize the importance of being present and responding thoughtfully to situations instead of reacting impulsively. Consider resilience as a muscle that gains strength through regular exercise; similarly, by consistently practicing self-care strategies such as setting achievable goals, seeking emotional support when necessary, and maintaining an optimistic attitude, you enhance your ability to handle stress and recover from difficulties more efficiently.

As we explore these facets of mental wellness, it becomes clear that the mind is not just a vessel to be filled, but a complex system to be nurtured and cared for. In the subsequent sections, we delve into the practical applications of these concepts, ensuring that you are equipped not only with the knowledge but also the tools to foster a resilient, healthy mind.

Emotional Wellness: Recognizing and Managing Emotions

At the core of holistic health, emotional wellness plays a pivotal role, yet it frequently slips under the radar amid our bustling lives. It's about acknowledging and valuing our emotions as crucial indicators that shed light on our overall health and shape how we interact with the world. Far from mere sentiments, emotions serve as essential alerts, signaling the state of our internal and external realms. They act as barometers for assessing the fulfillment of our needs and our connection to our surroundings. For instance, a continuous sense of sadness may suggest a longing for deeper relationships or more purposeful activities, whereas ongoing annoyance might point to overstretched limits, highlighting the need for firmer boundaries or the delegation of tasks.

This understanding leads us into the realm of emotional intelligence, a skill set that includes self-awareness, empathy, self-regulation, motivation, and social skills. Emotional intelligence profoundly impacts both personal and professional relationships, influencing how we communicate, resolve conflicts, and lead others. Self-awareness allows us to recognize our emotional triggers and understand their origins, which is the first step in managing them effectively. Empathy extends this awareness to others, enabling us to perceive and react to the emotions of those around us, thus fostering stronger and more harmonious relationships.

Managing our emotions, particularly intense ones such as anger or sadness requires practical strategies that can be seamlessly integrated into everyday life. Breathing exercises, for instance, are a powerful tool for regulating emotional responses. The simple act of taking deep, controlled breaths can activate the body's relaxation response, helping to calm the mind and reduce the intensity of emotional reactions. Mindfulness practices also play a crucial role in emotional regulation. By bringing our attention to the present moment and observing our thoughts and feelings without judgment, we can gain critical insights into the patterns of our emotional responses and develop greater mastery over them.

Cognitive reframing is another valuable technique in the emotional wellness toolkit. This strategy involves changing our perspective on a situation to alter its emotional impact. For example, viewing a stressful work project as an opportunity to develop new skills rather than a burden can significantly reduce feelings of anxiety and increase motivation. Real-life scenarios demonstrate the effectiveness of these techniques. Consider a professional faced with a daunting deadline. By practicing mindfulness, the individual can maintain focus and reduce panic, and by using cognitive reframing, they can transform anxiety into a driving force that enhances performance rather than a paralyzing fear.

These case studies not only highlight the practical applications of emotional wellness strategies but also underscore the transformative impact they can have on life outcomes and relationships. A person who masters emotional self-regulation is better equipped to handle interpersonal challenges, lead with confidence, and maintain a positive outlook in the face of adversity. This mastery does not come overnight but through consistent practice and a commitment to self-growth. By integrating these practices into our daily routines, we empower ourselves to lead more balanced, fulfilling lives, where emotions are not obstacles but valuable guides that lead us toward greater well-being.

Integrating Mindfulness into Everyday Life

Mindfulness, a term that's seen a surge in popularity but is often surrounded by misconceptions, is essentially about being fully present and engaged at the moment, aware of your thoughts and feelings without distraction or judgment. This practice,rooted deeply in Buddhist meditation, has been scientifically shown to modify the structures and functions of the brain, leading to improved mental clarity and reduced stress levels. Studies, like those published in the *Journal of Management*, indicate that mindfulness meditation can significantly decrease stress and enhance cognitive functions such as concentration, memory, and learning agility. Imagine the benefits of being less reactive to stressors at work or more attentive during conversations with loved ones. This isn't just about reducing stress; it's about enhancing the quality of every moment of your day.

Integrating mindfulness into daily activities can start with something as simple as mindful eating. This involves paying full attention to the experience of eating—observing the colors, smells, textures, and flavors of your food, and noticing the responses it evokes within your body. This practice not only enhances your enjoyment of meals but can also help regulate appetite and improve digestion. For instance, by eating mindfully, you might notice when you are full, reducing the likelihood of overeating. Similarly, mindful walking—where you focus intently on the movement of your body and the sensation of your feet touching the ground—can transform a routine walk to the subway into a revitalizing break from the mental chatter of your day.

Another practical way to incorporate mindfulness is during daily routines like showering or commuting. While showering, for instance, you can focus on the sensation of water on your skin, the sound of the water droplets, and the scent of your soap, turning a mundane activity into a refreshing ritual that clears your mind. If you commute, try turning off the car radio for a few minutes or put away your phone if you're on public transport. Use this time to breathe deeply and observe your surroundings, noting anything you can see, hear, or feel. This isn't just about 'killing time' but making the most of these moments to rejuvenate your mind.

In the workplace, mindfulness has proven its worth beyond just being a personal wellness tool; it enhances productivity and creativity. Incorporating mindfulness techniques like scheduled breathing breaks or a few minutes of guided meditation can help manage work-related stress, fostering a calmer mind that's better equipped to tackle complex tasks and brainstorm creative solutions. Research from the *Mindfulness Journal* suggests that mindfulness practices can reduce mental fatigue and burnout caused by multitasking and constant digital connectivity, common challenges in today's workplace settings.

By embedding mindfulness into the fabric of our daily lives, we not only improve our well-being but also bring greater attentiveness and care into our interactions with others. Whether it's through a deeper engagement with our work, more meaningful conversations with family, or simply enjoying a meal without the distraction of our screens, mindfulness offers a way to live richer, more fulfilled lives. The beauty of mindfulness lies in its simplicity and accessibility; it doesn't require special equipment or unusual skills, just a commitment to paying attention to the here and now. By embracing these practices, you can start to see significant changes, not just in your mental health, but in all aspects of your life, reinforcing the interconnectedness of your experiences and your wellness.

The Science of Stress and its Holistic Counteractions

Stress, a constant companion in both our professional and personal realms, has become a staple of modern life. At the heart of stress lies the body's ancient fight-or-flight mechanism, an instinctual response that unleashes a surge of hormones like cortisol and adrenaline to prepare us for immediate action. While this mechanism was crucial for survival in natural environments, it's less beneficial amidst the non-stop demands of today's world, such as endless emails and consecutive meetings. The very hormones that equip our forebears to evade predators persist in our bodies, leading to physical manifestations such as a faster heartbeat, elevated blood pressure, and a compromised immune system. This persistent state of alert not only depletes our bodily systems but also impacts our overall health, paving the way for a spectrum of issues including digestive disturbances and cardiovascular diseases.

Turning to holistic stress management, practices such as yoga and tai chi offer more than just a moment of calm. These ancient techniques stand out for their dual ability to soothe the mind and fortify the body. Yoga, with its series of postures and controlled breathing exercises, helps in reducing tension and enhancing blood circulation, which in turn lowers blood pressure and boosts mood. Similarly, tai chi, often described as meditation in motion, promotes serenity through gentle movements, reducing the body's stress responses and improving physical balance and stamina. Beyond these, herbal supplements like ashwagandha and lavender are lauded for their natural soothing properties that can help stabilize the body's cortisol levels, thus supporting the body's natural resilience against stress.

The fabric of community and social connections also plays a pivotal role in buffering against stress. Sociological studies have consistently shown that strong social networks enhance an individual's ability to manage stress and recover from illness more quickly. This support system can be as simple as having someone to talk through daily frustrations with or as involved as community groups that provide social interaction and collective problem-solving. Engaging with others can mitigate feelings of isolation and helplessness that often accompany high stress, providing not just emotional comfort but also practical assistance and advice. For instance, consider how a support group for new parents can alleviate the stress of child-rearing by offering a platform to share experiences, advice, and encouragement, reinforcing not only individual coping capacity but also fostering collective resilience.

However, the stakes of ignoring stress management are high. Chronic stress, if left unchecked, can lead to serious health issues such as cardiovascular diseases and mental disorders like depression and anxiety. These conditions not only diminish the quality of life but also place a burden on healthcare systems. Through holistic practices, which advocate for a preventative approach, the risks associated with prolonged stress can be significantly mitigated. Embracing a lifestyle that incorporates stress-management techniques, community support, and natural remedies not only enhances your immediate well-being but also sets the foundation for a healthier, more vibrant life.

Setting Realistic Wellness Goals That Resonate with Your Lifestyle

Embarking on a wellness journey that aligns with your life circumstances involves more than just temporary changes; it's about implementing changes that endure. Developing a personal wellness plan that addresses your physical, mental, emotional, and spiritual well-being is comparable to charting a map toward your optimal self. The challenge lies not only in plotting this course but also in crafting it to be practical and achievable within the complexities of your daily life.

Crafting a wellness plan is akin to nurturing a garden, requiring it to be customized to fit the unique dynamics of your life, whether that's the pace of your career or the demands of family life. Start by examining every aspect of your health. Set goals to increase physical activity or improve your diet, aim for better stress management and deepen connections with loved ones for mental and emotional well-being. For spiritual health, dedicate time to meditation or connecting with nature. The beauty of a holistic approach lies in understanding how improvements in one area can positively impact others. For instance, regular physical activity not only boosts heart health but also enhances mood and vitality through endorphin release, encouraging more social and spiritual engagement.

Setting goals is a craft in itself. They should be SMART—Specific, Measurable, Achievable, Relevant, and Time-bound. Specific goals dispel ambiguity, guiding you toward success with clarity. Measurable objectives enable progress tracking, offering a sense of accomplishment as you achieve milestones. Goals should be Achievable to avoid discouragement and sufficiently challenging to stimulate growth. They must also be Relevant to your broader life ambitions and Time-bound, with a realistic deadline for completion. For instance, instead of a vague aim to "eat healthier," a SMART goal could be "to incorporate two servings of vegetables into my dinner five nights a week for the next month." This approach not only integrates the goal into your routine but also ensures it's practical and measurable.

Life, however, is not static. It throws curveballs like a new job across the country, the birth of a child, or unexpected personal challenges. These changes can derail even the most well-thought-out wellness plan. The key is adaptability. When major life changes occur, take them as opportunities to reassess and adjust your goals. Perhaps after moving to a new city, your goal to jog in the local park every morning becomes impractical due to a longer commute. You might switch to weekend hikes or find a closer gym. The ability to pivot and reshape your wellness strategies around new circumstances is crucial. It ensures that your approach to health and wellness grows with you, reflecting your current realities rather than remaining a relic of your past.

Continuous learning and adaptation are key to evolving your wellness journey. As health trends shift and personal needs change, especially with aging, it's crucial to stay updated on wellness practices. This may involve transitioning from high-intensity workouts to gentler activities like yoga or incorporating mindfulness to ease career stress. Connecting with a supportive community, be it through local classes, online forums, or friend groups, enriches this journey with shared insights and encouragement. Ultimately, the aim is to develop a flexible wellness plan that fits your current lifestyle and future goals. Prioritizing health with this adaptable strategy enables you to face life's challenges head-on. A well-integrated wellness approach fosters habits that boost happiness and fulfillment.

> *"Holistic wellness begins with the foundation of nurturing the mind, body, and spirit, creating a balanced life that thrives on harmony and well-being."*

Chapter 1 Wellness Plan: Introduction to Holistic Wellness

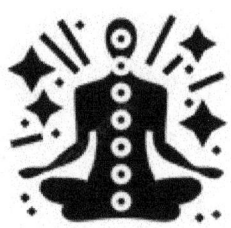

Activity: Setting Your Wellness Goals

Identify Your Goals

List three specific wellness goals you want to achieve (e.g., improve sleep quality, increase physical activity, reduce stress).

Daily Habits

Write down one daily habit you can adopt for each goal (e.g., go to bed at the same time every night, take a 20-minute walk, practice deep breathing).

Weekly Check-In

Schedule a time at the end of each week to reflect on your progress. Note any challenges and adjust your habits as needed.

Reflection Questions:

★ *What motivated you to choose these goals?*

★ *How do you feel when you make progress toward these goals?*

Meditation: Visualization (5 minutes)
★ *Sit comfortably and close your eyes.*
★ *Take a few deep breaths and relax your body.*
★*Visualize yourself achieving one of your wellness goals.*
★*Imagine the positive impact it has on your life and how you feel achieving it.*

Suggested Music:
★ **Ambient Music:** *Brian Eno's "Music for Airports"*
★ **Instrumental Guitar:** *Andy McKee's "Art of Motion"*

By regularly reflecting on your goals and progress, you can stay motivated and make meaningful strides toward holistic wellness. Use the visualization meditation to strengthen your commitment and envision the positive changes in your life.

Chapter 2

Nutrition for the Mind and Body

Imagine this: it's late afternoon, you're just finishing a hectic workday, and your energy levels are hitting a new low. We've all been there, right? Now, amid the chaos, reaching for that candy bar feels like a quick fix. But what if your desk drawer was stocked with nutrient-packed snacks that not only satisfy your hunger but also boost your energy and focus? This chapter is dedicated to transforming how you think about food, making nutrition an integral and effortless part of your busy lifestyle. Let's explore how a balanced diet can be your secret weapon for maintaining high energy, sharp focus, and overall well-being—even on your busiest days.

Balanced Diets for Busy Professionals: Quick and Nutritious Choices

The foundation of maintaining energy and focus throughout a demanding day lies in the power of balanced nutrition. But let's be real: when your schedule is packed, spending hours preparing complex meals isn't just impractical; it's nearly impossible. That's where the magic of quick-prep, nutritious foods comes into play. Foods like Greek yogurt with a handful of nuts, smoothies packed with fruits and vegetables, or whole-grain wraps filled with lean protein such as turkey or hummus are not only easy to prepare but are also incredibly nutrient-dense. These options provide a balanced mix of proteins, fats, and carbohydrates, which are essential for sustaining energy. For instance, starting your day with a smoothie that includes spinach, a banana, and a scoop of protein powder can keep you satiated and sharp for hours.

Now, let's talk about meal prepping, a strategy that can revolutionize your eating habits without burdening your schedule. The concept is simple: dedicate a few hours over the weekend to prepare large batches of meals that can be easily stored and quickly served throughout the week. Think of cooking a large tray of roasted vegetables, grilling several chicken breasts, or preparing a big pot of quinoa. These can then be mixed and matched to create different meals throughout the week, saving you a significant amount of time and decision-making each day. Moreover, embracing the use of healthy, ready-made options like pre-cut vegetables or canned beans can further streamline your meal preparation process, ensuring you always have the building blocks of a healthy meal at hand, even when time is not on your side.

Balancing macronutrients is another key aspect of a nutritionally sound diet, especially important when your days demand a lot from you. Proteins, fats, and carbohydrates play distinct and vital roles in your body. Proteins are essential for building and repairing tissues; fats provide a long-lasting source of energy and aid in nutrient absorption; carbohydrates, particularly complex ones like those found in whole grains, are your body's main energy source. Ensuring that each meal includes a balanced proportion of these macronutrients can help maintain your energy levels consistently throughout the day. For example, a lunch that includes a grilled chicken salad with mixed greens (proteins and fats from chicken and dressing), a whole-grain roll (carbohydrates), and some avocado slices (healthy fats) is balanced and will keep you full and focused well into the afternoon.

Lastly, let's not forget about the importance of snacks. Healthy snacks play a crucial role in bridging meals and keeping hunger at bay, which helps in maintaining focus and preventing overeating at meal times. Portable, easy-to-carry snacks such as almonds, carrots with hummus, or an apple with peanut butter provide a quick energy boost and essential nutrients without the added sugars and unhealthy fats found in typical vending machine fare. Keeping these healthy snacks within easy reach throughout your day ensures that you're never too far from a nutritious energy boost, helping you manage your hunger and maintain your focus until your next meal.

By integrating these straightforward and practical nutritional strategies into your daily routine, you can ensure that even on the busiest days, your body and mind are well-nourished, keeping you energized and focused from morning until night. Whether it's choosing the right kinds of foods, prepping meals in advance, balancing your intake of macronutrients, or snacking smartly, these habits can transform your approach to daily nutrition, making a balanced diet an achievable and essential part of your high-performance lifestyle.

Superfoods and Their Role in Mental Clarity

The term "superfood" has become a buzzword in the wellness community, often evoking images of exotic berries and rare seeds. But what exactly qualifies a food as a "superfood"? Essentially, superfoods are nutrient powerhouses that pack large doses of antioxidants, vitamins, and minerals. They offer more bang for your nutritional buck, providing enhanced benefits that can support overall health, including brain function. For instance, consider foods like blueberries, known for their high levels of flavonoids which have been shown to improve memory and cognitive function. Then there's salmon, rich in omega-3 fatty acids, crucial for brain health and maintaining sharp cognitive abilities as we age.

The nutritional content of these superfoods is what sets them apart. Take dark leafy greens such as spinach and kale, which are loaded with vitamins A, C, E, and K, along with fiber, iron, magnesium, potassium, and calcium. These nutrients contribute not only to physical health but also support brain function by enhancing blood flow and reducing inflammatory processes within the brain, which can cloud mental clarity. Similarly, nuts and seeds like walnuts and flaxseeds offer omega-3 fatty acids and antioxidants that combat oxidative stress and inflammation in the brain, factors that can affect focus and clarity.

Incorporating these nutrient-dense foods into your daily meals doesn't require a complete overhaul of your diet or advanced culinary skills. Start simple by adding a handful of spinach to your morning smoothie or topping your yogurt with a mix of berries and seeds for an afternoon snack. Swap out your usual side of fries for a vibrant salad packed with mixed greens, avocado, nuts, and a sprinkle of chia seeds to not only satisfy your hunger but also feed your brain. These small, manageable adjustments can make a significant impact on your mental clarity and overall health.

However, it's essential to approach the superfood trend with a balanced perspective. While these foods are indeed beneficial, they are not cure-alls and should be part of a varied and balanced diet. Myths abound, suggesting that superfoods can single-handedly prevent diseases or offer miraculous health benefits. It's crucial to debunk these myths and recognize that while superfoods are helpful, they are most effective when consumed as part of a broader healthy lifestyle that includes regular physical activity and adequate hydration. No single food holds the key to good health, but a smart combination of these nutrient-rich foods can certainly contribute to maintaining a sharp and focused mind amidst the demands of your busy life.

Managing Dietary Needs Without Stress

Navigating the world of nutrition can often feel like trying to solve a complex puzzle, especially when you factor in individual dietary needs and restrictions. Whether these are due to health conditions, allergies, or personal wellness goals, understanding and managing these requirements shouldn't add extra stress to your already busy life. Let's walk through how you can identify your specific dietary needs and create a plan that flexibly fits into your lifestyle, ensuring that you can enjoy meals without worry, even in social settings.

Identifying your unique dietary needs is the first step toward a more personalized and effective nutrition plan. Start by considering any known health conditions or allergies that directly impact your diet. Consulting with a healthcare provider or a dietitian can provide a solid foundation of what foods to embrace or avoid. For instance, if you have diabetes, understanding the types of foods that influence blood sugar levels is crucial. Beyond medical advice, paying attention to how your body reacts to different foods can also guide your choices. Perhaps you notice that dairy products make you feel sluggish or bloated, suggesting a possible lactose sensitivity. Keeping a food diary can be an insightful tool in this journey, helping you track your food intake and your body's reactions, simplifying the identification of foods that support or hinder your well-being.

Once you've pinned down your dietary needs, the next challenge is crafting a diet plan that is both flexible and forgiving, accommodating the unexpected twists of daily life. The goal here is to create a framework that allows for adjustments without compromising nutritional balance or adding to your stress levels. Start by building a list of 'safe' foods that you know are good for you and that you enjoy eating. From this list, you can create a variety of mix-and-match meal options that can be quickly adapted based on your daily schedule and availability of ingredients. For example, if you're avoiding gluten, stocking up on gluten-free grains like quinoa and rice allows you to rotate your staples without mealtime becoming monotonous. Additionally, embracing the practice of batch cooking once or twice a week can ensure that you always have a base of healthy meals ready to go, which you can then tweak with different spices or fresh ingredients for variety.

In today's tech-driven world, numerous apps and resources can significantly simplify the task of tracking dietary intake and managing nutritional goals. Apps like MyFitnessPal or Yazio offer platforms where you can log daily meals and monitor your intake of macros and micronutrients, ensuring you stay on track with your dietary needs. These tools often come with customizable options where you can set reminders for meal times, water intake, and even grocery shopping lists that align with your dietary plans. This digital support not only aids in maintaining a consistent diet but also alleviates the mental load of having to remember every detail, allowing you to focus more on enjoying your food and less on managing it.

Handling dietary restrictions in social settings is often a concern for many, but it doesn't have to be a source of anxiety. When dining out, reviewing menus online beforehand or calling the restaurant to discuss your dietary needs can help ensure that there are suitable options for you, preventing any uncomfortable situations at the table. When attending social gatherings, offering to bring a dish that meets your dietary requirements can be a great way to participate without feeling restricted. It also introduces others to your type of diet, which can be a wonderful opportunity for sharing lifestyle choices and recipes. Communicating openly with friends and family about your dietary needs not only helps in managing social dining occasions but also builds understanding and support within your social circles, making these interactions more enjoyable and less stressful.

By taking these thoughtful steps, you can navigate your dietary needs with confidence and ease. From understanding what your body needs, crafting a flexible eating plan, leveraging digital tools for meal management, to navigating social meals without stress, each strategy is designed to support your dietary journey, making it a seamless part of your life rather than a constant challenge. This way, you can focus more on the joys of eating and less on the worries of what's on your plate.

The Impact of Hydration on Physical and Mental Performance

Fueling our bodies and minds for peak performance extends beyond nutrition and exercise; hydration plays a pivotal role, yet it's often overlooked. Drinking sufficient water impacts everything from our stamina to mental sharpness. It's essential for the optimal function of every cell, organ, and tissue. Water not only lubricates our joints and regulates body temperature but also ensures the delivery of vital nutrients throughout our body. Crucially, it supports brain functions, powering thought and memory processes. Achieving proper hydration means our brain can function efficiently, enhancing clarity, speed, and efficiency.

Grasping the science behind hydration reveals its profound effects on both body and mind, fundamentally altering how we view this everyday act. Hydration directly influences brain function and size; even slight dehydration can diminish cognitive abilities, complicate tasks and decision-making, and impair memory functions. A study in the Journal of Nutrition underscored that dehydration might result in attention deficits, slowed motor responses, and a heightened sense of difficulty in tasks.

Recognizing the importance of hydration, it's essential to personalize your daily water intake. Factors such as activity level, health status, and climate play a crucial role in determining your needs. Guidelines suggest about 3.7 liters for men and 2.7 liters for women as a baseline, inclusive of all fluids and food sources. However, these figures should be adjusted based on your physical activity and the environment you're in. It's important to attune to your body's signals, as they are the most reliable indicators of your hydration requirements.

Hydration significantly influences cognitive performance, enhancing focus and memory retention. This is crucial for tasks demanding high concentration, from important presentations to daily work routines. Research in the Human Brain Mapping Journal demonstrates that adequately hydrated individuals show more efficient brain function, particularly in areas related to planning and problem-solving. This efficiency not only boosts professional productivity but also enriches personal life, making the simple act of drinking water a powerful tool for improving mental agility and overall performance.

So, how can you ensure adequate hydration throughout the day? It's not just about drinking eight glasses of water. Innovations in how we consume water can make hydration an enjoyable and refreshing part of your daily routine. Infusing water with fruits, vegetables, or herbs is a fantastic way to enhance its flavor naturally, making it more appealing if you find plain water too bland. Try combinations like cucumber and mint or berries and lemon for a refreshing twist. These infusions not only make the water taste better but also add vitamins and antioxidants, boosting your nutrient intake. Another method is to set regular reminders on your phone or computer, prompting you to take hydration breaks. This can be especially useful if you tend to lose track of time during busy workdays.

Embracing these hydration strategies can significantly boost your physical stamina and mental acuity. Understanding the critical importance of water for both your body and mind, and finding creative methods to meet your hydration needs, turns the simple act of drinking water into a seamless and powerful tool for enhancing your overall health and well-being.

Planning Meals for Energy and Focus

When it comes to maintaining high energy levels and sharp focus throughout your bustling day, what you eat, when you eat, and how you balance your nutrients play pivotal roles. Let's break down the strategies and types of food that can transform your meal planning from a routine chore to a powerful tool for boosting your daily productivity and mental clarity.

Starting with the right foods is crucial. Certain items are known not just for their nutritional value but for their ability to enhance energy and concentration. For example, oats are a fantastic breakfast choice due to their high fiber content, which provides a steady release of energy into your bloodstream. This avoids the mid-morning crash that more sugary breakfast options can cause. Pairing oats with a protein source like Greek yogurt or a handful of nuts can further enhance their energy-stabilizing effect. Similarly, leafy greens such as spinach and kale are packed with iron, an essential mineral that helps in energy production and oxygen circulation in the blood. A lack of iron can lead to fatigue and reduced cognitive function. Including these greens in a lunchtime salad or smoothie can help keep your energy levels optimal.

Timing your meals can also significantly impact your energy and focus. The goal is to prevent the large spikes and dips in blood sugar levels that not only lead to energy crashes but also affect your concentration and productivity. Eating smaller, more frequent meals is a strategy that works well for many. For instance, instead of three large meals, breaking your food intake into five or six smaller meals can keep your metabolism active and maintain steady blood sugar levels. This could look like having a mid-morning snack of almonds and a banana between breakfast and lunch, followed by a mid-afternoon snack of hummus and carrots before dinner. This strategy can be particularly effective if your lifestyle includes irregular hours or high physical activity, as it provides continuous energy and helps in muscle recovery and repair.

Incorporating slow-release energy foods into your diet is another key strategy. Foods that are high in complex carbohydrates, such as whole grains, legumes, and starchy vegetables, provide a slower and more sustained release of energy.

This is due to their complex structures, which take longer to break down during digestion, providing a gradual supply of glucose into your bloodstream. For someone who has long days either at the office or managing home responsibilities, integrating these foods can prevent the lethargy that often hits mid-afternoon. A lunch that includes quinoa, chickpeas, and a variety of vegetables dressed with olive oil provides a balanced mix of complex carbohydrates, protein, and healthy fats, keeping you satiated and focused into the evening.

Let's put all this together into a sample meal plan that balances energy intake across the day, tailored to a typical busy lifestyle. Imagine starting your day with a breakfast of overnight oats prepared with almond milk, and chia seeds, and topped with fresh berries. This meal kicks off your day with a rich mix of fiber, protein, and antioxidants. Mid-morning, you could snack on a small handful of nuts to keep your energy up until lunch. For lunch, a quinoa salad with mixed greens, sliced avocado, and grilled chicken offers a perfect combo of complex carbs, healthy fats, and protein. Come mid-afternoon, when energy levels might typically start to wane, a green smoothie can give you a quick, nutrient-packed pick-me-up without the heaviness of more solid food. Finally, a dinner of grilled salmon with sweet potato and steamed broccoli rounds out the day with a meal high in omega-3 fatty acids, complex carbs, and essential nutrients, supporting both your brain function and overall health.

By understanding and implementing these principles of energy-boosting foods, optimal meal timing, and the incorporation of slow-release energy foods, your meal planning can effectively support both your energy levels and cognitive function, making every meal a step toward a more energetic and focused you.

Integrating Nutritional Strategies with Family Dining

Bringing balanced nutrition into the heart of family life not only enriches the dining table but also fosters lifelong healthy eating habits for everyone, from the smallest to the eldest. The challenge, of course, lies in preparing meals that cater to diverse tastes and nutritional needs without chaining you to the kitchen all day. Let's start with some family-friendly healthy recipes that are as nutritious as they are delectable, and designed to appeal to all age groups. For instance, a one-pan dish like baked salmon with a side of roasted carrots and potatoes can be a hit. It's rich in omega-3 fatty acids, beta-carotene, and essential minerals, covering a broad spectrum of nutritional needs while keeping the cooking and cleaning minimal.

Educating children about nutrition is another vital component. It's about making mealtime both fun and informative, turning it into an opportunity for kids to learn about what's on their plate. Why not let them be 'chef for a day'? With supervision, kids can help with simple tasks like rinsing veggies or mixing ingredients. During these activities, chat about the benefits of each ingredient, like how tomatoes are full of vitamin C, which helps keep their immune system strong. This not only helps children understand the value of good food but also makes them more likely to eat what they've helped prepare.

Dealing with different dietary preferences in a single household can be quite the tightrope walk. However, it's entirely possible to satisfy various palates and requirements without having to cook multiple distinct meals. Start by preparing versatile base dishes that can be customized according to individual preferences. For example, a vegetarian stir-fry can be served as is for those avoiding meat, or you can quickly sauté some chicken on the side for the carnivores in the family. This approach keeps everyone's taste buds happy and ensures that meal preparation remains straightforward and stress-free.

Encouraging healthy eating habits within the family setting goes beyond just serving nutritious meals. It involves creating a dining environment that promotes a positive attitude towards food. Regular family meals are a fantastic way to model healthy eating behaviors. When children see their parents enjoying a variety of foods, they are more likely to emulate those choices. Moreover, use mealtime as a chance to disconnect from screens and connect with each other. This not only improves digestion but also strengthens family bonds, making meals a nurturing experience for the body and soul.

In integrating these nutritional strategies into your family dining, you're doing more than just feeding the body; you're nurturing a foundation of wellness that can support your loved ones throughout their lives. By offering balanced meals, educating young ones about nutrition, accommodating various dietary needs, and fostering healthy eating habits, you turn the family table into a place of health, joy, and connection.

In wrapping up this exploration of family-focused nutrition, remember that the goal is to create a supportive eating environment that respects individual needs while promoting collective health. The strategies discussed here are designed not just to nourish but to inspire, bringing a sense of well-being that extends beyond the dinner table and into every aspect of life. As we close this chapter and move forward, the focus will shift to another crucial aspect of holistic health that often goes unnoticed—sleep. The next chapter will delve into how quality sleep is not just a pillar of good health but a foundation for vitality and well-being, exploring strategies to enhance sleep quality for you and your family.

"Proper nutrition fuels both the mind and body, creating a foundation for overall well-being and vitality."

Chapter 2 Wellness Plan: Nutrition for the Mind and Body

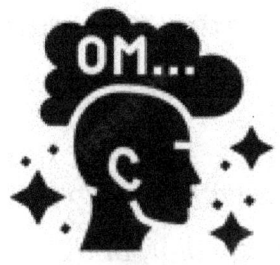

Activity: Daily Nutrition Reflection

Morning
- ★ What did you have for breakfast?
- ★ How did it make you feel (energized, sluggish, satisfied)?

Midday
- ★ What did you have for lunch?
- ★ Did you include any fruits or vegetables?

★ How did it impact your focus and energy in the afternoon?

Evening

★ What did you have for dinner?
★ Did you balance your proteins, fats, and carbohydrates?
★ How did it affect your overall well-being?

Reflection Questions:

★ *Which meal made you feel the best and why?*
★ *What changes can you make to improve your daily nutrition?*

Meditation: Mindful Eating (5 minutes)

★ *Sit in a quiet place with a small, healthy snack (like an apple slice or a few nuts).*
★ *Take a few deep breaths to relax.*
★ *Observe the texture, color, and smell of your snack.*
★ *Take a small bite, chew slowly, and notice the flavors and sensations.*
★ *Reflect on how mindful eating can enhance your appreciation and enjoyment of food.*

Suggested Music:

★ **Classical Piano:** *Chopin's Nocturnes, Op. 9*
★ **Nature Sounds:** *Forest or ocean waves*

Take a few minutes each day to jot down your reflections and notice any patterns in how your food choices impact your energy and focus. Use meditation to cultivate a habit of mindful eating.

Chapter 3

Physical Fitness in a Busy World

Picture this: it's early morning, you've just wrapped up a brisk workout, and you're feeling more alive and ready to tackle the day than ever before. Sounds ideal, doesn't it? Yet, for many of us juggling the demands of work, family, and personal commitments, regularly fitting in exercise can seem like a lofty goal. However, what if the key isn't finding more time but rather making the most of the time you do have with a flexible, tailored fitness routine that evolves with your lifestyle? That's exactly what we're diving into in this chapter—creating a fitness plan that not only fits into your busy schedule but also sparks joy and boosts your energy levels, making it a sustainable part of your daily life.

Designing a Flexible Fitness Routine

Assessing Personal Fitness Goals

Begin by assessing what you hope to achieve through your fitness routine. Goals in fitness are as varied as the individuals setting them. You might aim to build strength, enhance cardiovascular health, lose weight, or simply maintain your current fitness level. It's important to align these goals with your overall lifestyle and health status. Consider factors like your work schedule, family responsibilities, and any health conditions that might influence the type of activities best suited for you. For instance, a high-intensity workout might be perfect for a single professional looking to blow off steam after a busy day at the office, whereas a parent juggling work and kids might find more success with shorter, more frequent workouts that can be easily paused and resumed.

Creating a Modular Workout Plan

Once you have your goals in place, the next step is to create a workout plan that's as flexible as your week might be unpredictable. This is where the concept of a modular workout plan comes into play. Think of your weekly exercise routine as a collection of building blocks, each block representing a different activity that can fit into various time slots throughout your week. For instance, you might have a 30-minute block for a quick run, a 20-minute block for a yoga session, and even shorter 10-minute blocks for full-body stretches or quick high-intensity interval training (HIIT) sessions. The key is to develop a variety of these blocks that can be mixed and matched depending on how much time you have on any given day. This approach not only keeps your routine flexible but also prevents boredom and burnout, as you're not stuck doing the same workout every day.

Variety and Enjoyment

Speaking of variety, it's crucial for keeping your fitness journey enjoyable and effective. Incorporating different types of activities not only keeps things interesting but also ensures that you're working different muscle groups and giving others time to rest and recover. This could mean cycling between cardiovascular exercises, strength training, flexibility workouts, and balance exercises. Each type of exercise offers unique benefits and keeps your body guessing, which can help to prevent plateaus in your fitness progress. Moreover, consider what activities you actually enjoy. If you love being outdoors, make sure to include outdoor jogs or cycling in your routine. If you prefer group settings, a weekly dance class or a sports team meet-up might be the ticket to sustaining your fitness motivation.

Technology Aids

In today's digital age, technology offers a plethora of tools that can help you plan and track your workouts effectively. Fitness apps like MyFitnessPal or Strava not only help you monitor your physical activities but also provide insights into your progress, offer new workout ideas, and even connect you with a community of like-minded individuals for that extra dose of motivation. Wearable devices such as fitness trackers and smartwatches can be particularly useful, tracking everything from your step count and heart rate to your sleep patterns and recovery needs. These devices make it easier to stay on top of your fitness goals and adjust your routine as needed based on real-time data about your body's performance and needs.

By dedicating time to evaluate your fitness objectives, crafting a workout regimen that embraces flexibility, and leveraging technology for guidance and tracking, you pave the way for a fitness routine that seamlessly aligns with your dynamic lifestyle. This strategy guarantees a fulfilling and enjoyable path towards physical wellness, intricately woven into the fabric of your daily routine. It empowers you to enjoy the fruits of robust health and energy, ensuring your well-being thrives amidst the demands of life.

Home Workouts That Fit Your Life

Turning your home into a gym might sound like a daunting task, especially if you're short on space or don't have specialized equipment. But it's surprisingly feasible to create effective workout areas within the confines of your living space, using what you already own. Let's explore how you can transform your living area into a flexible gym that accommodates your fitness routine, no matter the size of your home.

For those working with limited space, the key is to utilize multi-functional furniture and areas that can easily be converted into workout zones. A yoga mat can turn any small space into a spot for yoga or pilates, and when you're done, it rolls up and tucks away. If you're looking to do more strength training, using sturdy furniture like a heavy chair or a low, stable table can substitute for gym equipment. For example, chairs can be excellent props for performing tricep dips or incline push-ups. Even a wall can be invaluable for exercises like wall sits or for stabilizing during a standing yoga pose. The idea is to look at your home not just as a place of rest but as a potential dynamic gym that you can maneuver around and adapt based on your workout needs.

Bodyweight exercises are a fantastic way to build strength and endurance without any equipment. Exercises like push-ups, sit-ups, planks, and squats are classics for a reason—they work. But beyond these basics, there are variations that can keep your routine engaging and challenging. For instance, switching from a regular squat to a single-leg squat can dramatically increase the intensity of the workout, targeting different muscle groups and improving balance. Introducing a routine of bodyweight exercises can be done in sequences or circuits, providing cardiovascular benefits alongside strength training, all from the comfort of your living room or bedroom.

In the digital age, you're never exercising in isolation, even from home. A wealth of online resources, including HIIT, dance, yoga, and strength training classes, are available at your fingertips through platforms like Peloton and apps such as Nike Training Club. These digital platforms not only provide a variety of workout options but also foster a community, offering connection and motivation to keep you consistent and engaged. Whether a beginner needing direction or an advanced user craving new routines, these online classes cater to all fitness levels.

By reimagining your living space, incorporating bodyweight routines, utilizing online resources, and involving the whole family, staying fit at home becomes not just an achievable goal but a sustainable and enjoyable part of your daily routine. These strategies ensure that your journey to fitness is as flexible and integrated into your lifestyle as it is beneficial to your health and happiness, proving that you don't need a gym membership to stay in shape and feel great.

High-Intensity Interval Training (HIIT) for Time-Savers

Imagine squeezing the most out of every workout minute, maximizing your fitness results without having to spend hours at the gym. That's the core premise of High-Intensity Interval Training or HIIT, a training technique that combines short bursts of intense exercise with periods of rest or lower-intensity exercise. The beauty of HIIT lies in its efficiency, making it an ideal workout for those who find it challenging to carve out extensive daily time for exercise. This method leverages the power of intensity to deliver significant cardiovascular and metabolic benefits in less time than traditional workout regimes.

The structure of a HIIT workout is simple yet incredibly effective. It alternates between periods of pushing your body to its max and allowing brief recovery times. For example, a typical session might involve 30 seconds of sprinting followed by 30 seconds of walking; this cycle is then repeated several times. Each burst of strenuous activity ramps up the heart rate, pushing the cardiovascular system to tap into energy reserves through anaerobic breathing. This not only improves heart health but also boosts metabolism, encouraging the body to burn more calories not just during the workout, but also for hours after.

To get you started, here's a sample HIIT routine that can be completed in just about 20-30 minutes and is adaptable to various fitness levels. Beginners might start with intervals of less intense activities like brisk walking alternated with moderate jogging. Those more advanced could opt for sprinting intervals interspersed with bodyweight exercises like squats or push-ups. Here's how you might structure it:

◆ Warm-up: 5 minutes of light jogging or a brisk walk to get your heart rate up.

◆ Cycle: 1 minute of sprinting followed by 1 minute of walking or light jogging, repeated 10 times.

◆ Cool down: 5 minutes of gradual slowing down of activity and stretching.

One of the most compelling benefits of HIIT is its ability to enhance cardiovascular health while effectively reducing body fat. The vigorous exertion required pushes the heart to pump faster, strengthening the cardiovascular system over time. Moreover, the intensity of the workout increases the metabolic rate, which means your body continues to burn calories at a higher rate even after you have finished exercising. This effect, known as the 'afterburn,' can be particularly beneficial for those looking to lose weight or improve their body composition.

Incorporating HIIT into your weekly routine can be seamlessly done, even with a tight schedule. Because these workouts are so efficient, you can fit them into various parts of your day. Morning person? Try a quick session first thing in the morning to kickstart your metabolism. More of a lunchtime exerciser? A 30-minute HIIT workout can be an excellent way to break up your day, leaving you energized for the afternoon. Even if your day is broken up with meetings or childcare responsibilities, HIIT's flexibility allows you to get a full workout in short, manageable segments, making it easier to maintain your fitness regimen without disrupting your daily responsibilities.

By embracing HIIT, you're not just saving time; you're also committing to a highly effective, scientifically backed method that enhances your health, accelerates fat loss, and boosts your endurance. Whether you're a busy professional, a parent managing a household, or someone simply looking to maximize their workout efficiency, HIIT offers a powerful solution to fit exceptional exercise into a compact time frame, ensuring you stay on track with your fitness goals regardless of your busy lifestyle.

The Role of Walking: Underrated Exercises

Walking, often overlooked in the rush for trendy high-intensity workouts or specialized fitness regimes, holds remarkable benefits for health that cater to all ages and fitness levels. Regular walking strengthens the heart, reduces the risk of cardiovascular disease, and helps manage weight by boosting the metabolism. Furthermore, it's an excellent mood enhancer; stepping out for a walk on a sunny day can significantly uplift your spirits thanks to the natural endorphins released during physical activity. The simplicity of walking, coupled with its profound impact on health, makes it an ideal, low-barrier entry point for anyone looking to improve their physical and mental well-being.

Incorporating more walking into your daily routine can be surprisingly straightforward and requires little adjustment to your existing schedule. If you commute to work, consider getting off a bus or train stop earlier and walking the rest of the way. Alternatively, if you drive, parking further away from your office can provide a good brisk walk that wakes you up before the workday starts and helps you decompress on your way home. Lunch breaks also offer a perfect opportunity; a quick 10-15 minute walk after eating not only aids digestion but also helps avoid the post-lunch energy dip. For those working from home, setting reminders to take brief walking breaks can be beneficial. These short bursts of activity not only break the monotony of prolonged sitting but also enhance circulation and mental alertness.

With today's digital tools, monitoring your walking achievements is effortless. Fitness trackers and smartphone apps track steps, distance, and calories, making it simple to set and achieve daily or weekly goals. These goals offer a clear sense of progress and accomplishment. Engaging in app-based challenges or with friends adds a fun, motivational aspect to your routine, encouraging you to remain dedicated and consistently push your boundaries.

To enhance your walking routine and keep it interesting, consider varying your routes and trying different walking techniques. Interval walking, which involves alternating between fast and moderate paces, can improve your cardiovascular health in a way that's similar to interval training. Adding weights, like a weighted vest or ankle weights, can increase the intensity of your walks, building strength and endurance. Choosing paths with varied elevations or terrains challenges different muscle groups, enhancing balance and flexibility. These simple changes can diversify your walking routine, amplifying its health benefits and making every step count.

Walking, often underrated, is a versatile physical activity accessible to all. It's an ideal choice for enhancing health gently, without the intensity of rigorous exercise regimes. Integrating walking into daily life, along with tools for tracking progress and diversifying routines, offers extensive health benefits. It keeps exercise interesting and manageable, regardless of your fitness level. Walking is the perfect low-impact step to enrich your wellness journey.

Combining Fitness with Family Time

Integrating fitness into family life not only strengthens the body but also the bonds between family members, creating shared experiences that are both healthy and joyful. Picture a sunny Saturday morning where instead of scrolling through phones, the entire family is out cycling through the park, laughing and racing each other, or perhaps an evening where everyone winds down with a friendly game of soccer in the backyard. These activities do more than just burn calories; they build memories and strengthen relationships. Activities like hiking, cycling, and playing sports are not only fantastic ways to get everyone moving but also opportunities for teaching teamwork, respect for nature, and the joy of living an active life.

The benefits of incorporating fitness activities that the whole family can participate in are immense. For children, these activities help instill a love of exercise from an early age, setting the foundation for healthy lifestyle habits. For adults, it's a way to model healthy behavior and stay active, which can be especially challenging given the demands of parenting and careers. Moreover, when families engage in physical activities together, they experience a unique type of bonding. This shared experience can enhance communication, foster mutual support, and provide a sense of accomplishment that strengthens familial ties. Additionally, regular physical activity has been shown to improve mental health and emotional well-being for all ages, reducing symptoms of anxiety and depression and elevating mood.

Scheduling regular physical activities for the family requires some creativity and flexibility, especially with varying schedules and interests. One effective strategy is to establish a routine that incorporates physical activity into the weekly schedule. This could be as simple as designating Sunday afternoons for family hiking trips or setting aside time every evening after dinner for a walk around the neighborhood. The key is consistency and making sure these activities are viewed as fun and enjoyable rather than another chore on the list. It can also be helpful to involve the whole family in the planning process, allowing each member to choose activities. This not only ensures that the activities align with everyone's interests but also increases the commitment level of all family members.

Leveraging family fitness time as a learning moment adds significant value. While hiking, for example, parents can introduce children to various plants and animals, seamlessly integrating a science lesson into the exercise. Sports activities can become practical lessons in fair play, teamwork, and resilience. Discussing the health advantages of these activities instills in children the importance of being active, fostering a lifelong positive outlook on health and fitness. These discussions not only enrich the family's wellness knowledge but also make the shared experience more enriching. Such moments are pivotal in building a resilient, health-conscious family unit, transforming fitness from an individual undertaking into a collective journey of joy and well-being.

Overcoming Common Physical Activity Barriers

When it comes to maintaining a regular exercise routine, it's not uncommon to hit a few roadblocks along the way. Whether it's the struggle to find time, waning motivation, or physical constraints, these barriers can often derail even the best-laid fitness plans. However, recognizing and understanding these obstacles is the first step toward overcoming them and achieving your fitness goals.

Identifying Personal Barriers

The first step in overcoming any obstacle is to identify it clearly. For many, time constraints are a major barrier, with days filled from morning to night with work, family duties, and social obligations leaving little room for exercise. Others might find that motivation ebbs and flows unpredictably, making it hard to stick to a routine. Physical limitations, whether due to an injury, chronic condition, or general fitness level, can also pose significant challenges. By pinpointing exactly what's holding you back, you can tailor your approach to tackle these specific issues head-on. For instance, if time is your biggest challenge, tracking how you spend your day might reveal hidden pockets of time that could be dedicated to physical activity.

Strategies to Overcome Barriers

Once you've identified your barriers, the next step is to develop strategies to navigate around them. Planning workouts ahead of time can be incredibly effective, especially for those who struggle with time management. At the start of each week, look at your schedule and block out times for physical activity, treating them as fixed appointments just like any other important commitment. For motivation issues, setting small, achievable milestones can help maintain a sense of progress and accomplishment. Celebrating these small victories can provide a continuous boost to your motivation levels. Additionally, finding a workout buddy or joining a fitness group can offer the necessary encouragement and accountability to keep you on track. The social aspect of exercising with others can transform your workout from a chore into an enjoyable social activity.

Adapting Exercises for Physical Limitations

For those dealing with physical limitations, adapting exercises to fit your abilities is key. Many exercises can be modified to accommodate different levels of mobility or strength. For example, if you have knee problems, you might switch from high-impact activities like running to lower-impact options such as swimming or cycling, which provide cardiovascular benefits without excessive strain on your joints. Resistance training can be adjusted by changing the weight, the number of repetitions, or even the speed of execution to better suit your capabilities. Consulting with a physical therapist or a certified fitness trainer who can provide personalized advice and modifications can ensure that you not only avoid injury but also make the most of your workout sessions.

<u>*Building a Support System*</u>

Finally, building a support system can play a crucial role in maintaining your motivation and commitment. This network can include friends, family, fitness professionals, or even online communities that share your fitness goals and challenges. Sharing your goals and progress with this group can make the journey less daunting and more supported. Whether it's having a friend to remind you of your workout appointments, family members who encourage you to stay on track, or a personal trainer who tailors your exercise program to your evolving needs, each component of your support system serves to keep you motivated and focused on your fitness goals.

By actively addressing each barrier with specific, tailored strategies, you can transform the way you approach physical activity. It becomes less about finding time or motivation and more about creating a lifestyle that naturally incorporates fitness into your daily routine. With each small step, whether it's a modified exercise to suit your physical condition or a quick workout squeezed into a busy day, you're building a foundation for lasting health and wellness that respects both your body's needs and your life's demands.

The Importance of Rest and Recovery

In the rhythm of push and pull that characterizes a well-rounded fitness regimen, the value of rest and recovery cannot be overstated. Often, the enthusiasm to achieve physical goals leads us to overlook these critical components, yet they are as vital as the workouts themselves. Rest days are essential in any fitness plan as they allow muscles to repair, rebuild, and strengthen. More importantly, they help prevent injuries that could otherwise set you back significantly. During high-intensity workouts, muscle fibers undergo stress and develop small tears. It's during the recovery period that these fibers heal and grow stronger, preparing your body to handle similar stress in the future more efficiently. This cycle of stress and recovery ultimately leads to physical improvements, making rest an indispensable part of training.

Recognizing the signs of overtraining is crucial in maintaining a healthy balance in your fitness journey. Symptoms like persistent muscle soreness, feeling drained instead of energized after a workout, insomnia, irritability, and a plateau or decline in performance can all indicate that your body needs more rest. These signals should not be ignored as they are your body's way of communicating that it cannot cope with the demands being placed on it. Listening to these signs and adjusting your training accordingly is essential to prevent burnout and injury. Remember, more is not always better; sometimes, the best thing you can do for your body is to allow it time to rest and recover.

Active recovery plays a pivotal role in any fitness routine by promoting recovery without overexertion. Techniques such as yoga, stretching, and light walking keep the body moving and blood circulating, which helps in reducing muscle stiffness and speeding up the healing process. Yoga, for instance, combines physical postures with breathwork and meditation, aiding in muscle and mental relaxation while improving flexibility and balance. Similarly, a gentle walk or a light cycle session can invigorate your muscles without the intensity of a full workout. These activities provide the benefits of keeping you physically active and engaged while still supporting the recovery process.

The deep connection between sleep and physical performance is essential. Quality sleep is crucial for recovery, as the body repairs muscles and releases growth hormones during deep sleep. To enhance sleep quality—and, consequently, recovery—try establishing a consistent bedtime, creating a quiet, dark sleeping environment, and avoiding caffeine before bed. Sleep-tracking apps can also help optimize your rest. Better sleep not only supports physical recovery but also boosts cognitive function and mood, enhancing your overall fitness journey.

Incorporating rest and recovery strategies, acknowledging signs of overtraining, engaging in active recovery, and prioritizing good sleep hygiene is crucial for a successful fitness regimen. They enable sustainable training, enhancing physical strength and overall well-being. As this chapter concludes, remember that rest days and recovery periods are as vital as the workouts themselves. Embracing this balance safeguards your health and propels you towards achieving your fitness goals with vitality and resilience.

As we transition from understanding the foundational elements of physical fitness, the focus will shift toward mental, emotional, and spiritual wellness in the upcoming chapters. These facets are intricately linked with our physical state and exploring them will provide a more holistic view of what it means to live a truly healthy life.

"Even in a busy world, physical fitness is essential; it nourishes the body, sharpens the mind, and enriches the spirit."

Chapter 3 Wellness Plan: Physical Fitness in a Busy World

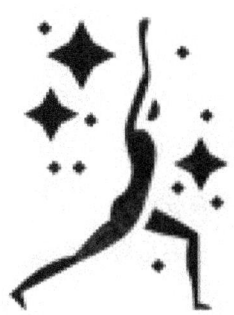

Activity: Reflective Exercise

Take a moment to reflect on your current approach to physical fitness in the context of your busy lifestyle. Consider the barriers you face, the strategies you've used to overcome them, and any areas where you feel there's room for improvement. Then, jot down your thoughts in a journal or notebook. Here are some prompts to guide your reflection:

1. **Identify Your Barriers:** *What are the main obstacles preventing you from maintaining a consistent fitness routine? Are they related to time, motivation, physical limitations, or something else entirely?*

2. **Strategies for Overcoming Barriers:** *Reflect on the strategies you've implemented to overcome these bar-*

riers. Which ones have been most effective for you? Are there any new approaches you'd like to try?

3. **Reflect on Progress:** Take stock of your progress so far. What achievements are you proud of? What challenges have you encountered, and how have you worked through them?

4. **Future Goals:** Based on your reflections, what are your goals for improving your physical fitness moving forward? How do you plan to integrate these goals into your busy lifestyle?

Music Suggestions:

★ **Energetic Playlist:** Curate a playlist of high-energy songs that get you pumped up and ready to tackle your workouts. Include upbeat tracks from your favorite artists or explore new genres to find tunes that inspire movement and motivation.

★ **Instrumental Relaxation:** Wind down after a workout or during moments of reflection with soothing instrumental music. Choose calming melodies or ambient sounds that promote relaxation and rejuvenation, helping you recharge for the next phase of your journey.

Once you've completed your reflection and chosen your music selections, take a moment to acknowledge the effort you've put into prioritizing your health and well-being. Remember, progress is a journey, and every step forward, no matter how small, is a victory worth celebrating.

Chapter 4

Mental, Emotional, and Spiritual Health Nourishment

Imagine your mind as a serene landscape, where thoughts flow like a gentle river, emotions bloom like vibrant flowers, and your spirit soars like the wind above. Sounds idyllic, doesn't it? Yet, for many of us, this mental landscape often feels more like a stormy sea than a tranquil garden. The challenges of balancing demanding careers, family responsibilities, and personal aspirations can stir up stress, anxiety, and a host of emotional upheavals. However, nurturing your mental, emotional, and spiritual health is as crucial as maintaining your physical well-being—perhaps even more so, as it forms the core from which our overall health radiates. This chapter is dedicated to equipping you with practical, accessible strategies to cultivate a resilient, peaceful mind and a nourished spirit, transforming your mental landscape into the serene haven you envision.

Practical Mindfulness Exercises for Anxiety

Breathing Techniques

One of the most immediate ways to temper anxiety is through mindful breathing, which can shift your body's response to stress from a state of alarm to one of calm. Techniques like the 4-7-8 breathing method, developed by Dr. Andrew Weil, are particularly effective. Here's how you do it: breathe in quietly through your nose for 4 seconds, hold your breath for 7 seconds, and exhale forcefully through your mouth, pursing your lips and making a "whoosh" sound, for 8 seconds. This method serves as a natural tranquilizer for the nervous system, slowing your heart rate and calming your mind. Another powerful technique is box breathing, used by Navy SEALs to stay calm and focused. It involves inhaling to a count of four, holding your breath for four seconds, exhaling for four seconds, and holding again for four seconds, forming a box pattern. Practicing these breathing exercises daily, or whenever anxiety begins to creep in, can help you regain control of your emotions, grounding you in the present moment.

Mindful Observation

When anxiety levels rise, turning your focus outward can help diminish their grip. Mindful observation involves selecting any object in your immediate environment and noting every detail about it. It could be a tree you pass by every day, a book on your coffee table, or simply a cup of coffee. Observe the colors, textures, shapes, and even the way light interacts with the object. This practice helps anchor your mind in the now, diverting it from anxious thoughts about the past or future, and fostering a serene attentiveness that can refresh and reset your emotional state.

Guided Visualizations

Guided visualizations are a form of mental escape that can provide powerful relief from anxiety. By mentally transporting yourself to a peaceful setting—say, a quiet beach at sunset or a cool, dark forest—you engage your mind in creating calming sensations that can overpower anxious thoughts. You can find guided visualization scripts online or through meditation apps like Calm or Headspace, which guide you through scenic narratives designed to engage your senses and transport you to tranquility.

Mindfulness Meditation

Integrating simple mindfulness meditation into your daily routine can significantly enhance your ability to manage anxiety. This practice involves sitting quietly and paying attention to your thoughts, breathing, or sensations in your body without judgment. Every time your mind wanders, gently bring it back to your focus point—be it your breath, a word, or a phrase. The key is consistency; even five to ten minutes a day can make a profound difference. Over time, mindfulness meditation increases your awareness of the present moment, allowing you to catch anxious thoughts before they spiral and address them with a calm, centered mind.

Through these practical exercises—breathing techniques, mindful observation, guided visualizations, and mindfulness meditation—you can cultivate a toolkit that empowers you to navigate the ebbs and flows of mental and emotional tides with grace and resilience. The beauty of these practices lies in their simplicity and accessibility, making it possible for anyone, regardless of their hectic schedule or life demands, to integrate them into daily life, paving the way toward a more peaceful, mindful existence. As we continue to explore the various dimensions of mental, emotional, and spiritual wellness, remember that each step you take on this path enriches not just your own life but also the lives of those around you, creating ripples of positivity and health that extend far beyond the immediate.

Cognitive Behavioral Techniques Without the Jargon

Identifying Cognitive Distortions

Navigating the maze of your thoughts can sometimes feel like a daunting task, especially when negative thinking patterns begin to cloud your judgment. Cognitive distortions, simply put, are ways that our mind convinces us of something that isn't really true. These inaccurate thoughts usually reinforce negative thinking or emotions, telling us things that sound rational and accurate, but really only serve to keep us feeling bad about ourselves. For instance, 'all-or-nothing' thinking leads you to view everything at extremes with no middle ground, while 'catastrophizing' involves expecting the worst-case scenario to happen. Recognizing these patterns is the first step in managing them. When you catch yourself thinking "I didn't finish this project perfectly, I'm a failure," that's all-or-nothing thinking. Start by simply noticing these thoughts and labeling them. This awareness creates a mental space between you and your reactions, providing a moment to choose how you respond.

Challenging Negative Thoughts

Once you identify these distortions, the next step is to challenge and reframe them into more balanced thoughts.

This is where you question the validity of your negative thoughts and replace them with more positive and accurate ones. It's like being a detective examining the evidence for and against your established way of thinking. For example, if you're thinking, "I will never be good at this," ask yourself, "What evidence is there to support this?" Most likely, you'll find that there are past instances where you have succeeded or made significant improvements. By methodically disputing these negative thoughts, you gradually diminish their power over your emotions and begin to see a more realistic picture of yourself and your abilities.

Behavioral Activation

Behavioral activation is a tool for overcoming depression and anxiety by encouraging you to engage in activities that you find meaningful and enjoyable. It operates on the principle that doing pleasant activities, particularly those that align with your values, can improve your mood and reduce feelings of anxiety. Start by making a list of small activities that bring you joy or a sense of satisfaction. This could be anything from reading a book, taking a walk in nature, or playing a musical instrument. The key here is consistency and gradually increasing the frequency of these activities. Over time, as you engage more in these fulfilling activities, you'll likely find a shift in your mood and outlook, breaking the cycle of negativity that feeds depression and anxiety.

Journaling for Cognitive Change

Journaling is a powerful tool for cognitive restructuring, offering a way to track your thoughts and patterns over time. By keeping a daily log of your feelings and the thoughts that accompany them, you begin to uncover patterns and triggers in your thinking. Use your journal to apply the cognitive techniques you've learned: write down distressing thoughts, identify the distortions, and challenge them. Over time, this practice can lead to significant shifts in how you perceive and react to the world around you. It's a personal reflection space where you can openly explore your emotions and the cognitive processes influencing them, fostering a deeper understanding and mastery over your mental health.

By employing cognitive behavioral techniques, you gain practical tools to transform your mental landscape. Identifying and correcting distorted thinking, engaging in activities that lift your mood, and journaling for reflection fosters a positive and fulfilling mental state. These strategies not only improve your mental and emotional health but also encourage proactive steps towards a more balanced lifestyle. As we delve deeper into mental and emotional wellness strategies, remember that each action you take is a step towards a clearer, more serene mind.

Building Resilience Against Daily Stressors

Developing a Resilience Mindset

In your daily life, stressors can range from small annoyances to large challenges. Developing a resilience mindset is like constructing a dam to control stress, preventing it from overwhelming you. It's not about dodging stress but learning to navigate through it. This mindset is built on acceptance, growth, and positivity. Acceptance means recognizing stress as an inevitable part of life, thereby reducing the tension that comes from resisting it. Growth involves viewing challenges as opportunities to learn and enhance your abilities, encouraging a proactive stance towards stress. Positivity, the third pillar, shapes your stress response, helping you find the good in situations, maintain high spirits, and adopt a problem-solving attitude.

Stress Inoculation Training

Stress Inoculation Training (SIT) is a technique designed to bolster your ability to manage stress by gradually exposing you to it in a safe, controlled way—similar to how vaccines build immunity. This method unfolds in three stages: understanding stress and your reactions to it, learning and practicing stress management skills like relaxation and positive thinking, and then applying these skills in increasingly challenging situations. For example, to conquer a fear of public speaking, you might begin by talking to yourself in the mirror, then move on to presenting in front of a small group of friends, and finally, speak at larger, more formal events. This step-by-step exposure helps diminish the anxiety and fear tied to stressors, thereby strengthening your resilience.

Routine Building

Creating a daily routine is a powerful strategy to mitigate stress by introducing structure and predictability into your life. By identifying the core elements of your day—such as meal times, work, exercise, and family interactions—and organizing your schedule around these, you decrease the mental burden of decision-making and the stress of unforeseen events. This structure provides a sense of control and efficiency, acting as a shield against stress. It's essential, however, to weave relaxation and leisure into this framework to ensure ongoing self-care and stress management. Additionally, a well-considered routine can stabilize your biological clock, leading to better sleep and higher energy levels. Remember, the essence of a beneficial routine lies in its flexibility; it should accommodate spontaneous needs and adjustments, preventing the rigidity from becoming a stressor itself.

Support Networks

The strength of a support network is invaluable in reducing stress. Comprising family, friends, colleagues, or support groups, it offers emotional solace and practical assistance when needed. Opening up to trusted individuals not only eases your emotional burden but also brings fresh perspectives and solutions. It counters the isolation stress often brings. Professionally, sharing tasks and solutions or just having someone who listens can be a significant relief. Building these connections demands mutual effort and trust, involving active participation in community events, clubs, or online groups, thereby broadening your support circle and fortifying your resilience.

These resilience-building strategies are crucial in your journey to holistic wellness. By cultivating a resilient mindset, engaging in Stress Inoculation Training, establishing a balanced daily routine, and fostering a robust support network, you empower yourself to navigate life's challenges more smoothly. These steps not only improve your current stress management but also arm you for future hurdles, promoting sustained health and fulfillment. As we delve deeper into mental, emotional, and spiritual wellness, remember that these strategies are interconnected, each enhancing the other towards a harmonious and enriched life.

Managing Social Anxiety Through Small Steps

Navigating social landscapes can often stir a whirlpool of anxiety for many, turning simple interactions into daunting challenges. If you find yourself feeling tense before a social event or rehearsing conversations in your mind long after they've ended, you're not alone. Tackling social anxiety doesn't have to be an overwhelming leap; small, manageable steps can significantly ease the journey, making social interactions less intimidating and more enjoyable. Let's explore some gentle yet effective strategies designed to help you build confidence and reduce anxiety in social settings.

Gradual Exposure

    The concept of gradual exposure is a cornerstone in managing social anxiety. It involves slowly and systematically confronting social situations that you find anxiety-inducing, rather than avoiding them. Start with less challenging interactions, such as saying hello to a neighbor or asking a store clerk a question, and gradually work your way up to more anxiety-provoking scenarios like attending a large gathering or giving a presentation. Each exposure opportunity allows you to experience and handle anxiety in a controlled manner, which over time, can help diminish the intensity of your reactions to these situations. It's like dipping your toes in the water before diving in; each step builds your confidence and reduces the fear associated with social interactions.

Social Skills Training

Improving your social skills can also play a significant role in alleviating social anxiety. Basic training in this area might include learning effective conversation starters or practicing active listening skills. For starters, try commenting on a shared situation or environment, like remarking on the weather or a piece of artwork at an event. This not only breaks the ice but also provides a mutual topic for discussion. Active listening, where you focus fully on the speaker, nodding and responding appropriately, can help you engage more deeply in conversations, making interactions more meaningful and less stressful. These skills don't just ease anxiety; they enhance your ability to connect with others, enriching your social experiences.

Role-playing Exercises

Role-playing is another invaluable tool in your arsenal against social anxiety. It allows you to rehearse social scenarios in a safe, non-threatening environment, typically with a therapist or a trusted friend. By simulating a social interaction and practicing your responses, you can gain confidence and reduce anxiety about real-life encounters. For instance, role-playing a job interview with a friend can help you practice answers to common questions, reducing anxiety when you face the actual situation. Over time, these rehearsals can help desensitize you to the stressors of social interactions, making them feel more manageable and less intimidating.

Self-Compassion Exercises

Cultivating self-compassion is crucial, especially when dealing with anxiety in socially challenging situations. Practice exercises that foster kindness and understanding toward yourself, particularly when you feel you've fallen short in social interactions. One effective method is to write yourself a letter from the perspective of a compassionate friend. In this letter, address yourself with kindness, acknowledge your feelings, and offer encouragement. This exercise helps shift your perspective, reducing self-criticism and fostering a gentler, more forgiving view of your social performances.

Professional Help

Lastly, if social anxiety significantly impacts your ability to function in professional or personal settings, seeking professional help can be a vital step. Therapists specializing in anxiety disorders can provide guidance and support through proven techniques like Cognitive Behavioral Therapy (CBT) or Acceptance and Commitment Therapy (ACT). These therapies offer structured approaches to understanding and managing your anxiety, providing tools and strategies that are tailored to your specific needs. Additionally, support groups for social anxiety can also be beneficial, offering a platform to share experiences and learn from others facing similar challenges.

By approaching social anxiety with these small, structured steps—gradual exposure, social skills enhancement, role-playing, self-compassion practices, and professional guidance—you can navigate social landscapes with increasing ease and confidence. Each step not only builds your social skills but also reinforces your ability to manage anxiety, transforming daunting social interactions into opportunities for connection and growth. As you continue to apply these techniques, remember that progress in managing social anxiety is a gradual journey, marked by small victories and continuous learning. Each effort you make is a building block in constructing a more confident, socially engaged version of yourself, paving the way for richer, more fulfilling interactions.

Enhancing Sleep Quality for Emotional Well-being

Understanding how closely sleep is intertwined with your emotional and mental health can be a game-changer in managing stress and enhancing your overall life satisfaction. It's a two-way street: just as emotional stress can lead to sleep disturbances, poor sleep can exacerbate stress, creating a cycle that can be hard to break. Deep, restorative sleep, on the other hand, acts much like a reset button for the brain, allowing you to process emotional experiences and regulate mood more effectively. During the REM (Rapid Eye Movement) stage of sleep, your brain actively processes and consolidates emotions and memories from the day. If sleep is cut short or frequently interrupted, you miss out on this critical processing time, which can lead to more pronounced emotional reactions and a decreased ability to cope with stress. Moreover, a lack of adequate sleep is linked to a higher risk of conditions such as depression and anxiety. Prioritizing good sleep is not just about physical rest—it's about giving your brain the chance to heal, reset, and strengthen.

Sleep Hygiene Practices

Establishing effective sleep hygiene is key to improving your sleep quality. Consider sleep hygiene as the foundation of good sleep practices. A consistent sleep schedule is vital—aim to go to bed and wake up at the same time daily, reinforcing your natural sleep-wake cycle. Equally important is a pre-sleep routine to calm your mind, such as reading, taking a warm bath, or engaging in gentle yoga or deep breathing exercises. Creating a sleep-friendly environment is also crucial. Your bedroom should be a haven for rest: ensure it's comfortable, quiet, dark, and kept at a cooler temperature. Quality bedding and the use of blackout curtains or an eye mask can further enhance your sleep setting.

Tools for Better Sleep

In our modern, tech-savvy era, leveraging tools and technologies can greatly enhance sleep quality. Wearable devices like Fitbit and apps like Sleep Cycle offer insights into your sleep habits by monitoring movements and heart rate to track sleep stages, including REM sleep. This information allows for personalized adjustments to improve sleep patterns. Additionally, white noise machines can create a tranquil environment by emitting soothing sounds such as rain or ocean waves, masking external disturbances and promoting uninterrupted sleep.

Addressing Common Sleep Disturbances

Many people grapple with sleep disturbances stemming from stress-induced insomnia and disruptive environmental conditions. Techniques aimed at calming the mind, such as progressive muscle relaxation—which involves tensing and then relaxing muscle groups—and mindfulness meditation, can significantly mitigate the mental unrest that hampers sleep. Furthermore, addressing environmental disruptors is essential. Ensuring your sleep haven is dim, quiet, and cool, with the ideal temperature around 65 degrees Fahrenheit, can profoundly enhance sleep quality. Incorporating blackout curtains and white noise machines also helps in creating an optimal sleep environment conducive to restful nights.

By embracing these practices and tools—maintaining consistent sleep patterns, creating a conducive sleep environment, using technology to enhance sleep quality, and addressing common disturbances—you can significantly improve your sleep quality. This, in turn, supports your emotional and mental health, making it easier to manage daily stresses and maintain a balanced mood. As we continue to explore more aspects of mental, emotional, and spiritual well-being, remember that sleep is not just a period of inactivity; it's an active and vital process of renewal and healing, crucial for a vibrant, joyful life.

Tech Tools That Aid Mental Wellness

In an era where technology permeates almost every aspect of our lives, it's no surprise that it also offers tools to help manage our mental wellness. These innovations come in various forms, from apps that ease the symptoms of anxiety to wearable devices that help monitor our physiological states. Embracing these tools can provide a significant boost to managing everyday mental health challenges, making psychological well-being more accessible and manageable, especially for those balancing busy schedules.

Mental health apps, such as Headspace and Calm, are revolutionizing the way we manage stress and anxiety through guided meditations and sessions tailored to various needs and schedules. These platforms, including Moodpath, offer mood tracking and daily check-ins to monitor your emotional well-being, helping to identify patterns or triggers. Incorporating these apps into your routine—starting with a few minutes of meditation each morning, for instance—can significantly improve your emotional stability and set a positive tone for your day.

Wearable technology, such as Fitbit and Apple Watch, significantly aids mental wellness by monitoring heart rate variability (HRV), a crucial stress and emotional arousal indicator. These devices track your physiological state, enhancing your awareness of stress levels and suggesting when to pause for calming activities. For instance, an elevated heart rate signal could prompt you to take a moment for deep breathing or a brief walk. This immediate feedback is essential for effective stress management, allowing timely interventions to prevent overwhelming situations.

The rise of online therapy platforms like BetterHelp and Talkspace has dramatically increased access to professional counseling. These services offer text, voice, or video calls, making mental health support more convenient for those with hectic schedules or limited access to local services. With a wide selection of therapists, these platforms cater to a variety of needs, enhancing the accessibility and flexibility of receiving guidance for minor to moderate mental health issues. Virtual Reality (VR) technology presents a fresh approach to managing phobias and anxiety disorders. It simulates fear-triggering scenarios in a safe, controlled environment, allowing individuals to face their fears with a therapist's support. For example, VR can mimic flight experiences for those with a fear of flying, enabling them to practice coping strategies safely. The immersive quality of VR offers a unique and effective form of exposure therapy, serving as a practical alternative to facing fears in real life. With its growing accessibility, VR holds significant promise for personalized mental health interventions, marking an innovative step forward in therapeutic practices.

By integrating these technological tools into your mental health care strategy—whether through apps, wearable devices, online therapy, or VR—you can enhance your ability to manage stress, anxiety, and other mental health challenges more effectively. These tools offer practical, accessible solutions that fit into your lifestyle, empowering you to take control of your mental wellness in a way that feels tailored and responsive to your needs. As we continue to navigate the complexities of modern life, these technologies serve as valuable allies in our quest for mental and emotional balance, making the journey a little smoother and the load a little lighter.

Art and Music Therapy: Creative Outlets for Stress Relief

Engaging in art and music can be profoundly therapeutic, serving not only as outlets for creativity but also as effective tools for stress relief and emotional management. The act of creating art or enjoying music stimulates the release of endorphins, the body's natural feel-good chemicals, promoting relaxation and joy while reducing stress and anxiety. This process can help elevate your mood, boost your self-esteem, and provide a sense of accomplishment. Whether you're painting, drawing, playing an instrument, or just listening to your favorite tunes, the arts offer a unique pathway to tranquility and emotional balance that can be especially beneficial in today's fast-paced, often stressful environment.

Getting Started with Art Therapy

For those new to art as a form of therapy, the beginning can be as simple as grabbing a piece of paper and some colored pencils. Art therapy isn't about creating masterpieces; it's about expressing yourself and finding emotional release through the creative process. Start with simple activities like doodling or coloring in an adult coloring book. These activities don't require you to be artistically skilled but can provide a focus for your mind, drawing it away from stressors and allowing a meditative calmness to take over. If you feel more adventurous, try your hand at clay modeling or watercolor painting, which can be incredibly soothing and rewarding. Local community centers or art schools often offer classes that can provide structured guidance and introduce you to various materials and techniques. The key is to focus on the process rather than the outcome, letting your creativity flow freely without judgment.

Integrating Music into Daily Routine

Music's power to influence our emotions and mood is nearly universal, making it a fantastic tool for managing stress and enhancing well-being. To incorporate music into your daily life, consider creating playlists that resonate with different moods or activities. A playlist with calming, soothing tunes is perfect for unwinding after a stressful day, while an upbeat, energetic playlist can be motivating during a workout or when tackling household chores. If you play an instrument, setting aside time each day to play can be not only an enjoyable skill to cultivate but also a powerful stress reliever. Even if you don't play an instrument, simply sitting back and actively listening to music, allowing yourself to fully experience and engage with the sounds, can be a therapeutic practice. It can help center your thoughts and calm your mind, much like meditation.

Case Studies and Success Stories

The transformative power of art and music therapy is supported by numerous success stories. For example, a young professional overcame burnout through painting, reconnecting with her passion for life and work. Similarly, a retired individual battling depression found solace and community through guitar lessons, which alleviated his loneliness. These examples underscore the dual benefits of art and music: they serve as effective forms of personal therapy and means of building connections, thereby boosting emotional well-being. Art and music therapy are not only accessible and enjoyable but also powerful ways to improve mental health and manage stress. Engaging in these creative practices can uplift your mood, foster personal growth, and enhance life satisfaction. As we conclude this chapter, we emphasize the importance of incorporating these creative outlets into our routine as part of a comprehensive approach to nurturing our mental, emotional, and spiritual health. The insights gained here pave the way for exploring more holistic wellness strategies in subsequent chapters, aiming for a balanced and fulfilling life.

> "Nourishing your mental, emotional, and spiritual health is the cornerstone of holistic wellness, fostering inner peace and balanced living."

Chapter 4 Wellness Plan: Emotional and Mental Wellness

Activity Reflective Exercise:
Mindfulness Reflection:

★ **Reflection:** Think about a recent moment when you felt emotionally or mentally balanced. What were you doing? How did it make you feel?

★ **Example:** "I felt very calm and content while taking a walk in the park last weekend. The fresh air and nature around me brought a sense of peace."

Embracing Positivity:

★ **Reflection:** Identify three positive affirmations that resonate with you and explain why they are meaningful.

★ **Example:** "I am resilient. This affirmation reminds me of my ability to overcome challenges and keep moving forward."

MENTAL, EMOTIONAL, AND SPIRITUAL HEALTH NOURISHMENT

Wellness Rituals:

★ **Reflection:** Describe a daily or weekly ritual that helps maintain your emotional and mental wellness. How does it contribute to your overall well-being?

★ **Example:** "Every morning, I spend 10 minutes journaling my thoughts and intentions for the day. It helps clear my mind and sets a positive tone."

Emotional Check-In:

★ **Reflection:** Conduct a quick emotional check-in. Rate your current emotional state on a scale from 1 to 10 and describe why you chose that number. What can you do to improve or maintain this state?

★ **Example:** "Today, I feel like a 7. I'm generally happy, but a bit stressed about work deadlines. Taking short breaks and practicing deep breathing could help reduce the stress."

Music Suggestions:

Energetic Playlist:

Create a playlist of high-energy songs that boost your mood and motivation. Include tracks that inspire you to move and feel positive.

★ **"Happy" by Pharrell Williams**
★ **"Uptown Funk" by Mark Ronson ft. Bruno Mars**
★ **"Can't Stop the Feeling!" by Justin Timberlake**

Instrumental Relaxation:

Wind down with soothing instrumental music that promotes relaxation and calm. Choose melodies that help you relax after a busy day.

★ "Weightless" by Marconi Union
★ "Clair de Lune" by Claude Debussy
★ "Ambient 1: Music for Airports" by Brian Eno

Acknowledge Your Effort:

Take a moment to acknowledge the effort you've put into prioritizing your emotional and mental well-being. Reflect on one thing you are proud of achieving in your wellness journey. Celebrate this progress, no matter how small it might seem. Remember, every step forward is a victory worth celebrating.

Chapter 5

Spiritual Growth and Personal Faith

Imagine starting your day not with the blare of an alarm and a mad dash to get ready, but with a moment of peace, a sacred ritual that grounds you and sets a serene tone for the challenges ahead. In a world that often values productivity over tranquility, dedicating time to nurture your spiritual self can seem like a luxury. However, integrating spiritual practices into your daily routine can profoundly impact your emotional resilience, mental clarity, and overall sense of well-being. This chapter invites you to explore simple yet profound daily practices that can enhance your spiritual growth and enrich your life's tapestry, no matter how hectic your schedule might seem.

Daily Practices for Spiritual Growth

Establishing a Morning Routine

Setting the tone for your day can significantly influence your mindset and productivity. Incorporating spiritual practices such as prayer, meditation, or reading spiritual texts each morning can provide a foundation of peace and purpose. Imagine this routine as your personal sanctuary time—undisturbed, quiet moments where you connect with something greater than the day's to-do list. This might look like spending a few minutes in meditation, reflecting on a passage from a spiritual book, or simply sitting in silence, savoring the stillness before the day unfolds. These practices aren't just about spiritual enlightenment; they're about setting a deliberate, mindful tone for your day, giving you a reservoir of calm to draw from when stress and challenges arise.

Gratitude Journaling

In the rush of daily responsibilities, it's easy to focus on what's going wrong or what's missing. Shifting this focus to gratitude can dramatically alter your perception, enhancing both your spiritual and emotional well-being. Maintaining a gratitude journal is a simple yet powerful practice to cultivate this mindset. Each day, take a few moments to write down things you are grateful for. These don't have to be grand revelations; often, it's the small comforts and joys—like a delicious cup of coffee, a child's laughter, or a comforting chat with a friend—that fill our lives with meaning. This practice trains your mind to recognize and appreciate these moments, enriching your life experience and elevating your spirit.

Mindful Breathing

Breathing, often an automatic action, becomes a potent spiritual tool when done with intention. Practicing deep diaphragmatic breathing—inhaling deeply through the nose to expand the abdomen, pausing, then exhaling slowly through the mouth or nose—can center your spirit, calm the mind, and anchor you in the present. This simple exercise reduces stress and restores clarity and composure, seamlessly integrating mindfulness into moments of stress or decision-making.

Incorporating Spirituality in Work and Relationships

Spirituality transcends the boundaries of solitary reflection, infusing every facet of our daily lives with depth and meaning. Introducing brief meditative breaks throughout the workday can rejuvenate your mental clarity and enhance concentration, transforming routine tasks into opportunities for mindfulness. Similarly, practicing attentive listening and presence during conversations with colleagues and loved ones not only fosters deeper connections but also promotes a mutual exchange of respect and understanding. By integrating spirituality into both mundane and meaningful activities, you create a life imbued with intention and awareness, thereby enriching your interactions in the professional sphere and personal relationships alike.

Meditation and Its Varieties: Finding What Fits

Meditation, often envisioned as a monk in serene silence on a mountain peak, is actually a versatile and widely accessible practice that can be adapted to fit into the bustling lives of anyone—from a busy CEO to a stay-at-home parent. The beauty of meditation lies in its diversity; numerous types cater to different preferences and objectives. Take mindfulness meditation, for example, which immerses you in the now, fostering an environment of mindfulness and acceptance. It's ideal for anyone eager to dial down stress levels and boost their focus. Conversely, transcendental meditation relies on mantra repetition to usher in profound relaxation and tranquility, making it a perfect fit for individuals in search of a more guided form of meditation.

Guided visualization is another form of meditation where you are led through a series of visualizations to promote relaxation and mental clarity. This type can be especially appealing if you find it challenging to focus or if you are a visual learner. Lastly, loving-kindness meditation focuses on developing feelings of compassion and love towards oneself and others. It's a powerful practice for fostering positivity and reducing negative emotions like anger and resentment. Each type of meditation offers unique benefits and can be a tool for personal growth and wellness, depending on what you feel you need most in your life.

Incorporating meditation into your life need not be time-consuming. A brief session of five to ten minutes each day can bring significant benefits. Optimal times for meditation include during your morning routine, on a lunch break, or just before sleep. For those commuting, guided audio meditations can turn travel time into a moment of restoration. The key to experiencing the full benefits of meditation lies in regular practice, making it a natural and impactful part of your daily health regimen.

Adopting a variety of meditation practices into your routine transcends basic relaxation and concentration techniques. It unlocks access to a profound toolkit for enhancing every facet of your existence. Whether your quest involves seeking serenity, mental clarity, a profound spiritual bond, or emotional resilience, meditation offers a tailored pathway to achieve your unique aspirations. Integrating meditation into your daily schedule transforms it from a mere activity to a cornerstone of your wellness journey. Embark on this exploration with an open heart and consistent effort, letting your personal affinities lead the way. This method cultivates a sense of equilibrium, peace, and a profound connection with the here and now.

The Role of Nature in Spiritual Wellness

Stepping outside, feeling the breeze on your face, hearing the rustle of leaves underfoot, and seeing the sunlight filter through the trees can transform an ordinary day into an extraordinary moment of connection with the natural world. The benefits of spending time in nature are not just physical; they extend deeply into our spiritual and psychological well-being. Nature has a unique ability to heal, soothe, and restore us, often just by our simply being present within it. Engaging with the natural environment can significantly lift our spirits, enhance mindfulness, and reduce stress. This connection is rooted in our very makeup; humans evolved in natural settings, and despite modern life's pull toward urban environments, our affinity for nature remains profound.

For those looking to deepen their spiritual connection through nature, several activities can foster this bond. Hiking, for instance, offers more than just physical exercise; it provides an opportunity to experience the quiet majesty of nature, which can be a profound spiritual experience. Each step taken on a forest trail can be a step deeper into mindfulness, where the mind is focused, the heart rate slows, and the hustle of daily life fades away. Gardening goes beyond simple beauty, serving as a meaningful path to self-care and growth. Planting each seed represents a commitment to what lies ahead, and the diligent nurturing of plants reflects the fostering of one's growth and patience.

Walking barefoot on grass, a practice known as "earthing" or "grounding," imbues the body with a natural tranquility, alleviating stress and enhancing well-being. This simple act of connecting physically with the earth is a powerful reminder of our bond to the natural world, offering an immediate sense of peace and groundedness. Such experiences underscore the profound impact nature has on our spiritual and psychological health, serving as a sanctuary away from the modern urban lifestyle.

Nature itself can be a profound teacher, offering lessons on resilience, change, and interconnectedness. Observing the natural cycles of growth, decay, and rebirth can provide deep insights into the nature of our own lives. For example, watching a river persistently flow towards the sea can teach us about perseverance and the importance of following our course. Witnessing a tree stand tall through the seasons, enduring storms, and basking in sunlight, can remind us of the strength and flexibility required to face life's various challenges. These lessons, when contemplated, can enhance our understanding of life and our place within it, enriching our spiritual journey.

Creating sacred spaces in natural settings can further enhance this connection. Whether it's a corner of your backyard, a spot under a favorite tree in a local park, or a quiet place by a nearby lake, these spaces can serve as sanctuaries for meditation, reflection, and connection. You might consider placing objects that hold personal significance in these spaces or creating altars with natural elements like stones, plants, and water. These acts of personalization make the space uniquely yours, a physical manifestation of your spiritual connections to nature. Spending time in your sacred space, surrounded by the elements of the natural world, can be incredibly restorative and uplifting.

In embracing the natural world as part of your spiritual practice, you open yourself to a wellspring of peace, clarity, and connectedness. These experiences in nature not only provide a respite from the stress of daily life but also deepen your spiritual existence, offering a broader perspective and a renewed sense of wonder and gratitude for the world around you. As you continue to explore and integrate these practices into your life, you may find that your time spent in nature becomes essential to your spiritual wellness, a vital part of your path to inner peace and fulfillment.

Creating a Personal Ritual for Spiritual Health

Rituals are the threads that weave the fabric of our spiritual lives, offering both a structure to navigate the chaos of daily living and a profound means to celebrate life's milestones, both big and small. In a world that often prizes spontaneity and flexibility, the deliberate and thoughtful nature of rituals can provide a comforting sense of stability and continuity. These sacred acts serve as anchors, grounding us in our beliefs and values amidst the ebbs and flows of life. Whether it's a simple morning routine of lighting a candle and setting intentions for the day, or a complex ceremony marking personal milestones like birthdays or anniversaries, rituals remind us of who we are and what matters most to us. They create a rhythm to our lives that nurtures our spiritual health and bolsters our resilience against the unpredictability of the world.

Creating personal rituals that resonate with your beliefs and needs doesn't require adherence to rigid rules or elaborate preparations; rather, it's about crafting meaningful practices that reflect your individuality and support your spiritual journey. Start by identifying moments in your life that you feel deserve recognition or need special attention—perhaps a time of transition, like starting a new job or moving to a new home, or moments that call for healing, such as recovering from illness or loss. Once you've pinpointed these moments, think about actions that hold significant spiritual or emotional weight for you. This could involve writing down affirmations, planting a tree, or even preparing a special meal. The key is to imbue these actions with intention and mindfulness, transforming them into powerful acts of ritual that celebrate or soothe the soul.

Choosing symbols or artifacts that carry personal significance can enhance the power of your rituals. These objects act as visual and tactile anchors for your intentions, imbuing your practice with depth and focus. For instance, a particular stone picked up from a place you feel connected to can serve as a symbol of strength or stability. Similarly, photographs of loved ones might represent love and connection, serving as focal points in rituals that honor relationships. The sounds used during your rituals—whether chants, prayers, music, or simple silence—can also significantly affect the atmosphere, helping to transport you to a state of deeper contemplation or celebration.

Sharing your personal rituals with a community can be profoundly enriching. It not only strengthens individual spiritual practices but also fosters a sense of shared experience and mutual support. Imagine a ritual where friends or family gather to share stories of gratitude, each person lighting a candle to symbolize their thanks. Such practices create bonds of understanding and empathy, reinforcing community ties and providing a collective strength that supports each member's spiritual growth. Engaging with others in ritual practice not only deepens relationships but also expands your own spiritual perspectives, allowing you to experience the diverse expressions of faith and spirituality within your community.

Faith Across Cultures: Universal Wellness Lessons

In the rich tapestry of global cultures, diverse spiritual traditions converge on common grounds—teachings of compassion, mindfulness, and forgiveness. These principles, deeply embedded in the doctrines of major world religions, form a universal blueprint for wellness that transcends geographical and cultural boundaries. For instance, Buddhism teaches the practice of mindfulness and loving-kindness to cultivate peace within oneself and towards others. Christianity emphasizes forgiveness and love, with the principle of treating others as one would like to be treated oneself. Similarly, Islam promotes compassion and mindfulness through daily prayers and the practice of Zakat, or charity, which fosters a sense of empathy and responsibility towards the less fortunate.

Delving into these foundational teachings enriches our comprehension and underscores our collective desire for connection and purpose. It unveils how, despite diverse rituals and expressions, the core of our moral and spiritual wellness is strikingly alike. Such insights are enlightening for those on spiritual paths or deepening their grasp of humanity and spirituality. By embracing these universal truths, we access a treasury of knowledge that fortifies well-being, applying age-old wisdom to contemporary life, thus enhancing our spiritual journey.

Appreciating the diversity of spiritual paths enriches your own spiritual journey. It opens up a myriad of perspectives and practices that can invigorate your faith or spiritual practice with new insights and methodologies. For example, engaging with the Islamic practice of daily reflection, or Muhasaba might inspire you to incorporate regular self-assessment into your spiritual routine. Alternatively, the Jewish tradition of Sabbath observance, a day dedicated entirely to rest and spiritual enrichment, could encourage you to define clear boundaries for work and relaxation, enhancing your work-life balance and spiritual growth.

These interfaith explorations foster not only personal growth but also a deeper social understanding, promoting tolerance and respect in increasingly multicultural societies. By learning about and respecting diverse religious practices, you contribute to a more empathetic world where spiritual diversity is celebrated as a strength rather than feared as a divide. This approach not only broadens your spiritual horizons but also models a pathway for others in your community, promoting a culture of mutual respect and curiosity.

Moreover, integrating elements from various faiths into your personal spiritual practice should be approached with sensitivity and respect. It's essential to engage with these elements authentically and considerately, ensuring that your adoption of foreign practices is both respectful and meaningful. Start by learning deeply about the context and significance of the practices you wish to adopt. Engage with communities and leaders within those faith traditions, seeking guidance and understanding to ensure that your practices honor their origins and intentions. This respectful integration enriches your spiritual life, not only with diverse practices but also with a profound respect and appreciation for the beliefs of others, fostering a personal spirituality that is both inclusive and expansive.

As you weave these interfaith insights and practices into your life, you create a mosaic of spiritual wellness that is both deeply personal and expansively global. This approach does not dilute your beliefs but rather deepens them, allowing you to stand firmly in your faith while reaching out with openness and respect to the myriad of ways humanity seeks and finds meaning. In doing so, you contribute to a world where spiritual diversity is seen as an invaluable resource for wisdom, peace, and deep, universal wellness.

The Benefits of Spiritual Retreats in Everyday Settings

Spiritual retreats serve as serene sanctuaries for deep reflection and rejuvenation, delivering profound impacts that surpass their peaceful surroundings. They grant a pause from the relentless pace of daily existence, inviting a journey into greater self-awareness and spiritual discovery. Engaging in these retreats can profoundly deepen your comprehension of your own identity and life's purpose, providing designated moments to step back from habitual activities and forge a closer connection with your core being. These immersive experiences often catalyze valuable revelations that propel personal development, emotional restoration, and a refreshed life orientation.

Exploring the different types of retreats can open up a world of tailored experiences that cater to your specific spiritual needs. Silent retreats, for example, emphasize the power of silence as a tool for deep meditation and self-reflection, allowing participants to turn their attention inward without the distraction of conversation. In contrast, meditation retreats focus on deepening participants' practice and understanding of meditation, often incorporating various techniques to aid spiritual growth and mental clarity. Yoga retreats offer a blend of physical and meditative practices that aim to harmonize body and mind, enhancing both physical health and spiritual well-being. Choosing the right retreat involves assessing your current spiritual needs and goals. For instance, if you're looking to find peace in times of stress, a silent retreat might provide the tranquil environment necessary for profound mental and emotional rest.

Creating mini-retreats at home is a practical way to incorporate the benefits of spiritual retreats into your daily life without the need to travel or take extended time off. Designating specific days or weekends for focused spiritual practices can create a retreat-like atmosphere in the comfort of your own home. This might involve turning off electronic devices, engaging in extended meditation sessions, or spending time in reflective reading and journaling. By setting aside dedicated time for these activities, you create sacred spaces and periods that allow for deep self-exploration and rejuvenation, mirroring the restorative experience of a traditional retreat.

Incorporating the serenity and revelations from retreat experiences into your routine is essential for sustained spiritual growth and fortitude. This may include adopting daily rituals that mirror the insights gained, such as engaging in morning meditations or setting aside time for introspection.

Chapter Conclusion

In this chapter, we explored the enriching world of spiritual growth through daily practices, diverse meditation techniques, and the transformative power of nature and personal rituals. Each section offered practical strategies to deepen your spiritual connections and enhance your overall well-being, emphasizing the importance of integrating these practices into everyday life. As we transition to the next chapter, we will build on these foundations, exploring holistic approaches to maintaining physical health, mental clarity, and emotional resilience, ensuring a balanced and fulfilling lifestyle.

> "True holistic wellness arises when spiritual growth intertwines with unwavering personal faith, creating a balanced and fulfilling life."

Chapter 5 Wellness Plan: Spiritual Growth and Personal Faith

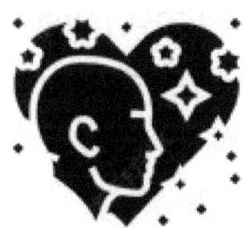

Activity Reflective Exercise:
Establishing a Morning Routine:
★ **Reflection:** Think about your current morning routine. How can you incorporate a simple spiritual practice to start your day with peace and purpose?

★ **Example:** "I will start my mornings with 10 minutes of meditation, focusing on my breath and setting positive intentions for the day."

Gratitude Journaling:
★ **Reflection:** Each day, write down three things you are grateful for. Consider how this practice impacts your spiritual and emotional well-being.

★ **Example:** "Today, I am grateful for the sunny weather, a kind gesture from a colleague, and a delicious meal."

Mindful Breathing:

★ **Reflection:** Practice mindful breathing for a few minutes each day. Reflect on how this practice helps center your spirit and calm your mind.

★ **Example:** "I noticed that mindful breathing helps me feel more present and reduces my anxiety, especially before important meetings."

Connecting with Nature:

★ **Reflection:** Spend time in nature and observe its beauty and tranquility. Reflect on how nature influences your spiritual growth and overall sense of well-being.

★ **Example:** "A walk in the park today made me feel connected to something larger than myself. The fresh air and sounds of nature brought me a sense of peace."

Creating Personal Rituals:

★ **Reflection:** Think about a personal ritual you can create that resonates with your spiritual beliefs and needs. It could be as simple as lighting a candle and setting an intention for the day.

★ **Example:** "I created a ritual of lighting a candle each evening and spending a few minutes in silent reflection. It helps me unwind and feel grounded."

Exploring Meditation Varieties:

★ **Reflection:** Try different forms of meditation, such as mindfulness, guided visualization, or loving-kindness meditation. Reflect on which type resonates most with you and why.

★ **Example:** "Guided visualization helps me relax and focus. I enjoy the creative aspect of imagining peaceful scenes."

Incorporating Spirituality in Daily Life:

★ **Reflection:** Think about how you can integrate spirituality into your work and relationships. Reflect on the impact this has on your interactions and overall well-being.

★ **Example:** "I started taking brief meditative breaks at work and noticed an increase in my concentration and a decrease in stress. Being present during conversations with loved ones has deepened my relationships."

Learning from Different Faiths:

★ **Reflection:** Explore spiritual teachings from different cultures and religions. Reflect on the universal lessons and how they can enhance your spiritual journey.

★ **Example:** "Learning about the concept of mindfulness from Buddhism has taught me to be more present and compassionate in my daily life."

Personalizing Your Spiritual Path:

★ **Reflection:** Reflect on the unique aspects of your spiritual journey. Consider how you can honor and celebrate these aspects through personalized practices and rituals.

★ **Example:** "I personalized my meditation space with objects that hold special meaning to me, making it a sanctuary for spiritual reflection."

Acknowledging Your Effort:

After completing your reflections and implementing new spiritual practices, take a moment to acknowledge your dedication to your spiritual growth. Celebrate the small steps you've taken and the progress you've made. Remember, spiritual growth is a continuous journey, and every effort counts towards a more fulfilling and balanced life.

Music Suggestions:
1. **Uplifting Playlist:**
    ★ "Higher Love" by Kygo & Whitney Houston
    ★ "Rise Up" by Andra Day
    ★ "Here Comes the Sun" by The Beatles
2. **Relaxing Instrumentals:**
    ★ "River Flows in You" by Yiruma
    ★ "Gymnopédie No. 1" by Erik Satie
    ★ "Morning Mood" by Edvard Grieg

End of Chapter Reflection:

Reflect on the various practices you've explored in this chapter. How have they contributed to your spiritual growth and personal faith? Consider how you will continue to integrate these practices into your daily routine and the impact they have had on your overall well-being. As you move forward, continue to explore and refine your spiritual practices, allowing them to evolve and grow with you.

By engaging in these reflective exercises and incorporating the suggested practices, you can deepen your spiritual growth and enhance your personal faith, leading to a more balanced and fulfilling life.

Chapter 6

Sustainable Living and Wellness

Imagine if every choice you made in your daily routine could contribute not just to your personal health, but also to a healthier planet. From the soap you use to wash your hands to the clothes you pick out of your closet, every decision has the power to impact both your well-being and the environment. In this chapter, we dive into the heart of sustainable living and wellness, exploring how making eco-friendly choices can lead to a life that's not only healthier for you but also kinder to the world around you. It's about transforming our everyday habits into actions that nurture our health and cherish the planet—an approach that aligns perfectly with the holistic wellness principles we cherish.

Eco-Friendly Choices That Enhance Personal Health

In today's market, shelves are stocked with products claiming myriad benefits, yet many of these benefits don't extend to the environment. Switching to biodegradable and natural personal care products, such as soaps, shampoos, and toothpaste, is a simple yet effective way to reduce your exposure to potentially harmful chemicals while also minimizing your ecological footprint. These products are crafted to break down more easily in the environment, preventing pollutants from accumulating in our ecosystems. Moreover, they are often made without harsh chemicals, reducing the risk of skin irritations, allergies, and other health issues that can arise from synthetic ingredients. By choosing these products, you're not just cleansing your body; you're contributing to a cleaner, healthier environment.

The clothes we wear and the goods we consume also play a significant role in sustainable wellness. Opting for clothing made from organic cotton or recycled polyester not only reduces environmental damage (like pesticide use and waste accumulation) but also supports industries striving to reduce their carbon footprint. Wearing a shirt made from organic cotton, you're supporting farming practices that maintain soil health and reduce toxic pesticide usage. Similarly, choosing consumer goods made from recycled or sustainable materials helps decrease the demand for raw materials, which often involve environmentally intensive extraction processes. These choices ensure that your personal wellness journey contributes positively to the health of the planet, aligning your lifestyle with your values of care and responsibility.

Transportation is another area where you can make significant eco-friendly changes. Opting for greener methods such as biking, walking, or using public transit not only reduces your reliance on fossil fuels but also benefits your physical health. Regular physical activity, such as biking to work, can improve cardiovascular health, enhance mental well-being, and decrease stress levels. Moreover, using public transit can help reduce traffic congestion and the pollution that comes with it, leading to cleaner air and a healthier community. These transportation choices are integral to a sustainable lifestyle, promoting both environmental health and personal well-being.

Lastly, reducing energy consumption in your home through energy-efficient appliances, LED lighting, and smart thermostats not only cuts down on your utility bills but also your carbon footprint. Energy-efficient appliances use less electricity, which means less fossil fuel is burned in power plants, leading to fewer air pollutants that can cause respiratory problems and other health issues. Smart therapeutics allow you to control your home's heating and cooling systems more efficiently, avoiding unnecessary energy use and promoting a healthier indoor environment. By making these adjustments, you contribute to a larger movement of energy conservation, which is crucial for our planet's health and our own.

Embracing these eco-friendly practices represents a powerful step towards living a life that values sustainability and wellness. It's about making choices that respect and renew our resources—choices that ensure we not only thrive but so does the world around us. As we continue to explore more ways to integrate sustainable practices into our daily lives, remember that each small change we make is part of a much larger process of transformation—one that promises a healthier, more sustainable future for all.

Reducing Your Carbon Footprint with Smarter Food Choices

Eating is an everyday activity that inevitably impacts the environment, but it also holds fantastic potential for positive change. By making mindful choices about what you eat and how you manage food, you can significantly reduce your carbon footprint while improving your health. Let's explore how adopting practices like local and seasonal eating, embracing a plant-based diet, reducing food waste, and supporting sustainable farming can transform your meals into a powerful tool for environmental conservation and personal wellness.

Local and seasonal eating is not just a trendy concept; it's one of the most effective ways to enhance the quality of your diet while minimizing environmental impact. Foods grown locally require far less transportation, which significantly reduces carbon emissions associated with long-distance food transport. Additionally, seasonal produce tends to be fresher and more nutrient-rich, as it is harvested at its peak and doesn't require long periods in storage, where nutrients can degrade. This means that the strawberries you buy from your local farmer's market in June are likely to be tastier and healthier than those shipped from halfway across the world in December. By choosing local and seasonal foods, you also support the local economy and small farmers who are more likely to use sustainable practices that maintain soil health and biodiversity.

Transitioning to a plant-based diet is another powerful way to lower your carbon footprint. Livestock production is one of the largest contributors to environmental degradation, including deforestation, water scarcity, and greenhouse gas emissions. By reducing your consumption of animal products, you can help decrease the demand for these resource-intensive foods. A plant-based diet, which emphasizes vegetables, fruits, grains, and nuts, is not only environmentally sustainable but also beneficial for your health.

Studies have shown that it can reduce the risk of chronic diseases such as heart disease, hypertension, diabetes, and certain types of cancer. Moreover, plant-based diets often encourage a more creative approach to cooking and eating, inspiring you to explore a wider variety of foods and culinary techniques.

Food waste is a massive global issue, with significant environmental, economic, and social impacts. In the United States alone, it is estimated that about 30-40% of the food supply is wasted. This not only wastes the resources used for growing, transporting, and selling food but also contributes to methane emissions from landfills, a potent greenhouse gas. You can combat food waste by planning your meals ahead, buying only what you need, and storing food properly to extend its freshness. Learning how to use leftovers creatively is another skill that can reduce waste while adding variety to your meals. For instance, yesterday's roasted chicken can be today's chicken salad, and wilting vegetables can be transformed into a nutritious soup or stock.

Supporting farms and businesses that adhere to sustainable practices is crucial in promoting an environmentally responsible food system. Organic farming, permaculture, and other sustainable agriculture methods not only help reduce environmental impact but also produce healthier, more nutritious food. These practices avoid or significantly reduce the use of synthetic pesticides and fertilizers, which can contaminate water, soil, and even the food itself. By choosing products from farms that prioritize sustainability, you help create demand for these practices, encouraging more farmers to consider environmentally friendly options. Many communities now have farmer's markets, community-supported agriculture (CSA) programs, and local health food stores that offer direct access to sustainably produced goods. By making these choices, you not only ensure healthier food for yourself and your family but also contribute to a larger movement towards a more sustainable and equitable food system.

Each of these strategies offers a pathway to reducing your environmental impact while enhancing your health and supporting your community. Whether it's through choosing local produce, adopting a plant-based diet, minimizing food waste, or supporting sustainable farming practices, the choices you make at the dining table can have a profound impact on the planet. As you continue to explore and implement these practices, you'll find that eating sustainably can also be a delicious, rewarding, and deeply fulfilling experience.

Sustainable Fitness: Environmentally Conscious Exercise

Embracing the great outdoors for your fitness regimen not only revitalizes your body but also deeply reconnects you with nature, enhancing both your physical well-being and mental clarity. Imagine starting your day with a hike through a lush forest trail, the sounds of nature replacing the hum of gym machines, or perhaps kayaking on a serene lake, where the rhythmic splash of your paddle sets a meditative pace. Outdoor activities like hiking, cycling, and kayaking don't rely on electric power, which diminishes your carbon footprint and immerses you in natural settings that promote significant health benefits. These activities increase your exposure to vitamin D, enhance your mood through natural scenery, and improve your physical fitness by engaging different muscle groups in a dynamic environment. The psychological benefits are just as impactful, with natural settings shown to reduce stress, enhance mood, and improve overall mental health.

Switching to eco-friendly fitness gear can further align your exercise routine with sustainable practices. Consider yoga mats made from natural rubber or pilates equipment crafted from recycled materials. These choices not only reduce your ecological impact but also ensure that your health pursuits contribute positively to the environment. Similarly, opting for workout clothing made from organic cotton or recycled fabrics can significantly reduce the demand for new fibers, which often involve resource-intensive production processes. These materials offer the same functionality and comfort as their non-eco-friendly counterparts, ensuring that your transition to sustainable fitness gear is seamless and beneficial.

The community aspect of sports can also play a pivotal role in promoting both environmental sustainability and social well-being. Participating in community sports leagues often makes use of local fields and facilities, which helps reduce the need for long commutes to distant venues, cutting down on carbon emissions. These community-based activities foster a sense of belonging and teamwork, enhancing your social connections while engaging in physical exercise. The shared experience of playing sports can lead to stronger community bonds and a collective commitment to maintaining local recreational areas, which further supports environmental conservation efforts.

Lastly, if you're looking to simplify your fitness routine while minimizing your environmental impact, consider minimalist workouts that require little to no equipment. Exercises like push-ups, sit-ups, squats, and jogging are not only highly effective but also accessible to everyone, regardless of their location or economic status. These activities can be performed anywhere, from the smallest apartment to a local park, making it easier to fit exercise into your busy schedule without contributing to consumer culture through the purchase of equipment. This approach not only helps in maintaining physical fitness but also ensures that your workout regimen is sustainable, affordable, and inclusive.

By integrating these environmentally conscious practices into your fitness routine—embracing outdoor activities, choosing eco-friendly gear, participating in community sports, and adopting minimalist workouts—you create a fitness lifestyle that not only benefits your health but also contributes positively to the well-being of our planet. Each step you take in this direction supports a sustainable future while empowering you to live a healthier, more connected life. As you continue to explore and implement these practices, you'll find that sustainable fitness is not only about personal health but also about nurturing a deep respect and care for the environment we all share.

Household Toxins and Natural Alternatives

When you think about maintaining a healthy home, what often comes to mind is a space that's clean, well-organized, and inviting. But beneath the surface of shiny floors and polished countertops, there could be unseen threats lurking in the form of household toxins. Common substances like

BPA, phthalates, and formaldehyde are found in a myriad of household products, from plastic containers to furniture and air fresheners. These chemicals are not just bad for the planet; they can pose significant risks to your health, including hormonal disruptions and an increased risk of cancer. Awareness and proactive management of these substances can transform your home into a truly safe sanctuary.

Switching to natural cleaning products is a straightforward and effective way to reduce your exposure to harmful chemicals. Many everyday pantry items can be powerful cleaning agents; for instance, white vinegar and baking soda can handle everything from window cleaning to unclogging drains and polishing silver. For a simple all-purpose cleaner, mix equal parts of water and vinegar in a spray bottle and use it to wipe down surfaces — it's effective, safe, and economical. Adding a few drops of essential oils like lemon or lavender can provide a pleasant scent along with additional antibacterial properties. These natural alternatives not only keep your home clean but also ensure that you are not inhaling harmful chemical residues that can affect your health.

Maintaining good indoor air quality is crucial for a healthy home environment, especially considering how much time most people spend indoors. Regular use of salt lamps and beeswax candles can help in reducing airborne contaminants. Salt lamps attract and neutralize positively charged contaminants, improving air quality, while beeswax candles burn cleanly and emit negative ions that can bind with toxins and help remove them from the air. Additionally, incorporating air-purifying plants such as spider plants, snake plants, and peace lilies can bring a touch of nature indoors while filtering out pollutants and releasing oxygen.

Dealing with pests without resorting to harsh chemicals can be a challenge, but natural methods like diatomaceous earth, neem oil, and peppermint oil offer effective, non-toxic alternatives. Diatomaceous earth is a powder made from fossilized algae that is deadly to insects but harmless to humans and pets; it can be sprinkled in areas where bugs are a problem. Neem oil, derived from the seeds of the neem tree, works as a natural pesticide that disrupts the life cycle of pests without harming beneficial insects like bees and butterflies. Peppermint oil, aside from its pleasant scent, is a potent repellent for many types of insects, including spiders and ants. A few drops in water can be used to make a spray that, when applied to entry points, can keep your home pest-free naturally.

By identifying and mitigating common household toxins through natural cleaning products, improving indoor air quality, and using natural pest control methods, you can significantly enhance both your health and your environment. Each small change you make contributes to a healthier home and a healthier planet, aligning your lifestyle more closely with holistic wellness principles. As you continue to explore more ways to integrate natural alternatives into your daily routine, remember that each choice you make builds toward a safer, cleaner living space that nurtures both the body and the Earth.

The Wellness Benefits of Minimalism

The allure of a minimalist lifestyle is often portrayed in images of pristine living spaces bathed in white and sparse furnishings that promise a calm, uncluttered existence. But beyond aesthetics, adopting a minimalist approach can profoundly impact your mental health and overall well-being. Consider the experience of coming home to a cluttered space, where every surface is covered with unsorted mail, items from past shopping trips, and half-done projects. This visual chaos can trigger stress and anxiety, making it hard to find peace or focus. Now, imagine entering a space that contains only what you need and love—where there's room to breathe and space to relax. This environment can significantly decrease stress and anxiety levels, enhancing your ability to focus and process information more effectively.

The concept of conscious consumption, a cornerstone of minimalism, advocates for buying less but choosing well. It's about prioritizing quality over quantity, which naturally leads to less waste and a more sustainable lifestyle. This practice not only helps in reducing the clutter that can overwhelm your home and mind but also aligns your purchasing habits with your values, leading to a deeper sense of satisfaction and purpose. When you choose to buy a well-made product that lasts longer, you're not just making a purchase; you're making a statement about the kind of world you want to live in—one that values sustainability over disposability. This mindful approach to consumption can significantly reduce the environmental impact of your lifestyle, supporting a healthier planet as well as a more focused and value-driven personal life.

Creating minimalist living spaces is about more than discarding unwanted items; it's about designing environments that promote peace and functionality. Start by identifying the essentials, the items that serve a purpose or bring you joy, and let go of duplicates and those that no longer serve you. This doesn't mean your space has to be bare; rather, it should be curated thoughtfully to support your daily activities and personal aesthetics. For example, a bedroom might only have a bed, a wardrobe, and a couple of meaningful decorations that promote a restful ambiance. Such spaces are easier to maintain and clean, which reduces the time and stress associated with household chores, leaving more time for activities that enhance your well-being.

Digital minimalism is another facet of this lifestyle that can lead to significant improvements in mental and emotional health. In an age where digital clutter is as overwhelming as physical clutter, learning to streamline your digital engagement can free up time and reduce stress. Start by unsubscribing from emails that no longer serve you and limiting your exposure to social media, which can be a major source of anxiety and distraction. Instead, allocate time to digital activities that add value, such as educational podcasts or meaningful conversations with friends and family online. This approach helps reclaim your time and mental space from the demands of a constantly connected world, allowing for deeper engagement with the real world and a more balanced, fulfilling life.

Embracing minimalism in these various forms creates a lifestyle that is not only sustainable but also conducive to a deeper sense of peace and contentedness. It's about making more room for the things that truly matter—whether that's relationships, hobbies, or personal growth—and shedding the excess that distracts from these priorities. As you continue to explore and implement minimalist practices, you'll likely discover that this less-is-more philosophy isn't just about giving things up. It's about creating space for growth, peace, and fulfillment in ways that resonate with your personal values and lifestyle, enhancing both your well-being and the world around you.

Community Gardening and Local Food Sources

Embracing the concept of community gardening and supporting local food sources is not just about cultivating plants; it's about nurturing a community and fostering a connection to the earth that feeds us. Imagine stepping into a lush community garden, where every plot and plant tells a story of collaboration and care. Here, local residents, each with their own unique backgrounds and experiences, come together to sow seeds not only of vegetables and flowers but of friendship and mutual support. The benefits of participating in such a community initiative extend far beyond the harvest of fresh produce. They also include significant boosts to physical activity, as gardening is a wonderfully gentle yet effective form of exercise. Additionally, the mental health benefits are profound—gardening is known to reduce stress and promote feelings of well-being.

Starting a community garden might seem like a daunting task, but it can be broken down into manageable steps. First, securing a piece of land is crucial. This space could be a vacant lot, a rooftop, or even a series of large containers in a shared space. Once a location is secured, engaging community members is the next step. This involves reaching out to local residents, schools, and organizations to garner support and participation. Choosing what to plant can be a community decision as well, one that might depend on the local climate, the soil quality, and the preferences of the community gardeners. It's also essential to consider the maintenance and sustainability of the garden, which includes regular watering, weeding, and harvesting schedules that volunteers can sign up for. By breaking down the process and involving the community at every step, the garden becomes a collective endeavor where everyone's input and effort are valued.

Local food co-ops offer another avenue for supporting local farmers and accessing fresh, seasonal produce. In a food co-op, members buy shares of a farm's harvest in advance, providing farmers with the upfront funds needed to cover initial production costs. In return, members receive a regular share of the harvest throughout the farming season. This model not only ensures that farmers have a guaranteed market for their produce but also allows consumers to become intimately connected with the source of their food, often receiving items that are fresher and more varied than what's available in supermarkets. Moreover, many co-ops provide opportunities for members to visit the farms, meet the farmers, and even participate in farming activities, offering deeper insights into the food production process and fostering a greater appreciation for the labor and love that goes into growing food.

Community gardens and local food sources also serve as exceptional educational tools. They provide hands-on learning opportunities for people of all ages, teaching valuable skills in gardening, nutrition, and environmental stewardship. For children, participating in a community garden can be an enlightening experience, one that teaches them where food comes from and the importance of taking care of the environment. Adults, too, can learn a great deal about sustainable gardening techniques, seasonal food patterns, and the nutritional benefits of fresh produce. Furthermore, community gardens can host workshops and events focused on topics such as composting, plant identification, and cooking with garden-fresh ingredients, enhancing the educational benefits for all involved.

As this chapter on community gardens and local food sources concludes, reflect on how integrating these practices into your life might not only change the way you eat but also how you connect with others and engage with your environment. These initiatives offer a pathway to a more sustainable lifestyle, one that promotes health, supports local economies, and strengthens community ties.

As we move forward, the principles and practices explored here can serve as a foundation for a broader discussion on sustainable living, one that encompasses not only our food choices but also our daily habits and consumer behaviors.

"Holistic wellness is the harmony we cultivate within ourselves and with the world around us, and sustainable living is the pathway to achieving this balance."

Chapter 6 Wellness Plan: Sustainable Living and Wellness

Activity: Practical Sustainability

Take practical steps towards integrating sustainable living and wellness into your daily routine. Reflect on each activity, document your experiences, and explore how music can enhance your journey.

Eco-Friendly Product Audit:

◆ List your current personal care and household cleaning products.

◆ Research eco-friendly alternatives.

◆ Purchase and try one eco-friendly product.

☆ **Reflection:**

☆ *How does the eco-friendly product compare to your usual one?*

☆ *What differences did you notice in effectiveness or sensory experience?*

Sustainable Wardrobe Update:
◆ Identify three clothing items to replace with sustainable alternatives.
◆ Research brands offering sustainable materials.
◆ Purchase one sustainable clothing item.
☆ **Reflection:**
☆ *How do you feel wearing the sustainable item?*
☆ *What did you learn about sustainable fashion?*

Greener Transportation Challenge:
◆ Use a green transportation method (walking, biking, public transit) for one day.
◆ Plan your route and schedule.
☆ **Reflection:**
☆ *How did green transportation affect your physical health and mood?*
☆ *What challenges did you encounter and overcome?*

Energy Efficiency Check:
◆ Audit your home's energy usage (lights, appliances, heating/cooling systems).
◆ Identify three ways to reduce energy consumption (e.g., switching to LED bulbs).

- Implement one change.

☆ **Reflection:**

☆ What changes did you make and how easy were they to implement?

☆ Did you notice any immediate differences in your home environment?

Plant-Based Meal Prep:

- Plan and prepare three plant-based meals using local and seasonal ingredients.

☆ **Reflection:**

☆ How did the plant-based meals make you feel?

☆ Did you enjoy the process of cooking and eating these meals?

Minimalist Home Detox:

- Choose one area to declutter.
- Sort items into categories: keep, donate, recycle, discard.
- Organize the space.

☆ **Reflection:**

☆ How did decluttering affect your mental and emotional state?

☆ Did the process reveal any insights about your consumption habits?

Join or Start a Community Garden:
- Research community gardens or start one with a group.
- Spend one hour this week gardening.

Reflection:
- *What benefits did you experience from gardening (physical, mental, social)?*
- *How did it enhance your connection to the community?*

Music Suggestions:
Energetic Playlist:
- *Curate a playlist of upbeat, motivational songs to energize you during eco-friendly product research or sustainable wardrobe updates. Include tracks that inspire action and positivity.*

Calming Tunes for Reflection:
- *Create a playlist of soothing instrumental music or ambient sounds to play during your minimalist home detox or plant-based meal prep. Use calming melodies to promote relaxation and mindfulness.*

Acknowledge Your Effort:
Take a moment to acknowledge the effort you've put into these activities. Reflect on the positive changes you've experienced and their impact on your health and the environment. Celebrate your progress and commit to continuing these sustainable practices.

Remember, every step towards sustainability and wellness is a victory worth celebrating. Keep moving forward and enjoy the journey!

Chapter 7

Social Wellness and Community Building

Imagine you're at a bustling coffee shop, surrounded by the chatter of friends catching up, colleagues discussing projects, and individuals deeply engrossed in books or laptops. This scene, vibrant with human connection, encapsulates the essence of social wellness—a fundamental aspect of holistic health that enriches our lives and buffers against the stresses of daily living. In this chapter, we delve into the art of building supportive relationships, a cornerstone of social wellness that not only enhances our emotional and mental well-being but also plays a critical role in our physical health and recovery processes.

Building Supportive Relationships

Understanding Support Systems

The value of a robust support system cannot be overstated. Psychologically, having a network of supportive relationships can significantly reduce stress, anxiety, and depression. Research consistently shows that individuals with strong social ties tend to live longer and experience better health outcomes. This phenomenon, often reflected in studies like those conducted by Julianne Holt-Lunstad at Brigham Young University, highlights that social connections can reduce mortality risk by up to 50%, underscoring the profound impact of our social environment on our longevity and vitality. These benefits are thought to arise because social support can buffer the physiological impacts of stress, and people within a supportive community often adopt healthier behaviors and feel a greater sense of purpose and belonging.

Cultivating Meaningful Connections

Developing these critical social ties means cultivating meaningful connections, both by deepening existing relationships and forming new ones. Active listening is a powerful tool in this endeavor. It involves fully concentrating on what is being said rather than passively hearing the message of the speaker. This practice helps build deeper, more empathetic connections, ensuring that your friends, family, and colleagues feel truly heard and valued. Shared activities also play a crucial role. Whether it's a weekly sports league, a book club, or a cooking class, engaging in regular communal activities can create a sense of camaraderie and commitment, strengthening bonds and providing regular social interaction which is key to building lasting relationships.

Navigating Challenges in Relationships

However, relationships aren't without their challenges. Conflicts and misunderstandings are inevitable, but the way we handle these situations can either strengthen or weaken our bonds. Effective communication skills are essential in navigating these waters. Techniques such as 'I' statements—expressing how you feel rather than accusing the other person—can foster understanding and prevent conflict escalation. Empathy also plays a crucial role; trying to see the situation from the other person's perspective can help resolve conflicts more amicably and maintain the strength of the relationship. Remember, the goal isn't to avoid all conflicts but to handle disagreements in ways that strengthen mutual understanding and respect.

Role of Support in Health Recovery

Support systems are particularly crucial during health challenges. Whether it's recovery from surgery, managing a chronic illness, or navigating mental health issues, having a network of supportive loved ones can significantly impact your recovery and ability to manage health conditions. They can offer practical help, like assisting with daily tasks or providing transportation to medical appointments, and emotional support, which can improve health outcomes. For instance, a study published in the *Journal of Clinical Oncology* found that breast cancer patients with robust social networks had significantly lower mortality rates and recurrence of cancer. These findings illuminate the powerful role that emotional support plays in the context of illness, highlighting how our social connections can quite literally be a lifeline during our most challenging moments.

Incorporating these aspects of building and maintaining supportive relationships into your life can transform your experience of the world. It enriches your emotional landscape, bolsters your mental resilience, and enhances your physical health. As you continue to weave these practices into the fabric of your daily life, you'll likely find that the quality of your relationships deepens, providing you with a stronger, more supportive network on which to lean, not just in times of need but every day. Engaging actively with this process of building and nurturing connections can turn each interaction into a meaningful exchange, enriching your life's tapestry with the threads of genuine relationships that support and uplift you through the complexities of life.

Communicating Needs and Boundaries

In the tapestry of daily interactions, whether with family, friends, or colleagues, the ability to effectively communicate your needs and set healthy boundaries is as crucial as any skill for maintaining your mental health and ensuring your relationships are both satisfying and supportive. Think about it this way: expressing your needs isn't just about getting what you want; it's about creating an environment where mutual understanding and respect flourish. This clarity helps prevent resentment and misunderstanding, which are often the root causes of relationship strain. For instance, clearly communicating your need for quiet time after work to decompress can help your family understand your actions and provide you with the space you need, thus avoiding feelings of neglect or irritation that might arise if you withdraw without explanation.

Setting boundaries is a natural extension of expressing your needs. It involves communicating to others what is acceptable and what is not, which helps manage their expectations and respects your limits. For instance, you might decide that you will not answer work calls during dinner time to ensure quality family time. It's important to convey these boundaries clearly and assertively, not apologetically. For example, you could say, "I value our team's hard work, but I won't be taking calls during dinner time to ensure I can recharge and be fully present for the next day's challenges." This kind of language not only sets a clear boundary but also communicates the value behind it, making it more likely to be respected.

Balancing self-care with caring for others is often a delicate dance, especially for those who naturally place others' needs before their own. The key here is to recognize that self-care is not selfish; rather, it's a prerequisite for effectively supporting others. Embracing the principle that one cannot give from an empty vessel is foundational to holistic wellness. Prioritizing your own needs ensures you are in the best position to support those you care about in a meaningful and sustained manner. This may involve dedicating moments for personal relaxation and rejuvenation before attending to the needs of others. Highlighting the significance of establishing personal boundaries, it's essential to understand that declining requests or asking for help as your energy depletes is not only acceptable but necessary. This practice not only protects your well-being but also sets a positive example, encouraging others to also treat their health with the same level of importance and care.

Dealing with pushback is often the most challenging aspect of setting boundaries. Not everyone will understand or respect your needs, and they may test your limits. It's crucial to stand firm in these situations and reiterate your boundaries with calm assertiveness. For example, if a family member repeatedly calls during your designated work hours, remind them of your availability with a gentle but firm reminder: "I understand you want to chat, which I love, but I need to focus on work during these hours. Can we schedule a call this evening instead?" If boundaries are continually disrespected, it might be necessary to seek external support, whether from other family members, friends, or a professional. This is not a failure but a proactive approach to maintaining your well-being and the health of your relationships.

Navigating the complexities of interpersonal dynamics through effective communication and boundary-setting is not just about avoiding conflict; it's about actively constructing a life that feels balanced, respectful, and fulfilling. As you improve in these areas, not only do your relationships deepen and become more satisfying, but your understanding of yourself and your needs becomes clearer. This clarity is empowering, enabling you to make choices that align more closely with your values and long-term well-being. As you continue to practice these skills, remember that each conversation is an opportunity to refine your approach and enhance your connections, making every interaction a stepping stone to a healthier, happier you.

Volunteering: The Health Benefits of Giving Back

When you lend a helping hand to others, the benefits extend far beyond the immediate impact of your actions. Engaging in volunteer activities can enrich your life in profound ways, boosting your emotional well-being and even enhancing your physical health. Think of it not just as giving back but as a key component of your holistic wellness strategy. Volunteering can infuse your life with a sense of purpose and fulfillment that is often hard to find in other pursuits. It's that heartwarming feeling you get when you see the direct impact of your efforts, whether you're helping to build a home, tutoring children, or planting trees in your community.

The emotional and psychological rewards of volunteering are immense. Engaging in altruistic activities can significantly boost your self-esteem and happiness. When you volunteer, you're often immersed in a supportive social environment that fosters positive interactions and teamwork. This social aspect can alleviate feelings of loneliness and depression by connecting you with others who share similar values and goals. Moreover, the act of helping others can give you a sense of purpose and satisfaction. A study from the London School of Economics found that people who volunteered were happier and felt they had better mental health compared to those who didn't. The researchers suggested that the personal rewards of volunteering are a vital component of the overall psychological benefits.

Volunteering also offers tangible physical health benefits. Regular volunteer work can significantly lower blood pressure, according to a study by Carnegie Mellon University, potentially reducing the risk of hypertension. This effect is thought to be connected to the stress-reducing properties of being helpful and working with others in a cooperative setting. Additionally, volunteering can increase longevity. A review of data from the Longitudinal Study of Aging found that those who volunteer have lower mortality rates than those who do not, even when controlling for physical health, age, and other factors. The physical activity involved in certain types of volunteer work can also contribute to better physical health, providing a low-stress workout environment that doesn't feel like exercise.

Finding the right volunteer opportunities is crucial in making sure that your efforts are as rewarding and impactful as possible. Start by identifying causes that resonate with your personal values and interests. Are you passionate about animal welfare, environmental conservation, or perhaps education? Once you've pinpointed areas you care about, look for organizations that work in those fields. Local nonprofits, religious groups, and community centers often have a variety of initiatives that could use help. When choosing a volunteering opportunity, consider how much time you can realistically commit. Some activities might require a regular weekly commitment, while others might be one-off events. By aligning your volunteering efforts with your personal values and time availability, you ensure that your experience is fulfilling and stress-free, allowing you to enjoy the emotional and physical benefits of your service fully.

Moreover, volunteering doesn't just benefit the individuals or communities being helped—it can also have a profound impact on the health of the broader community. Volunteers often bring energy and innovation to the organizations they work with, sparking improvements and inspiring others to contribute. This can lead to a more vibrant, active, and interconnected community. Furthermore, by addressing social issues and contributing to the common good, volunteering builds social capital, fostering stronger, more resilient communities that are better equipped to handle challenges and support their members. This interconnectedness of individual well-being and community health is a hallmark of the holistic approach to wellness, emphasizing that our health is deeply intertwined with the health of our social environment.

Group Fitness and Social Bonds

When you join a group fitness class or a sports league, you're signing up for more than just physical activity—you're stepping into a vibrant community of like-minded individuals who are there to motivate and uplift each other. The benefits of group exercise are manifold; not only does it enhance your physical fitness, but it also amplifies your motivation and enjoyment. Imagine the difference between jogging alone on a treadmill and participating in a lively group fitness class with upbeat music and enthusiastic companions. The energy in the room is contagious, pushing you to exert yourself more than you might have alone. This collective enthusiasm is a key element of group fitness that helps sustain participation over time, making your fitness journey a consistent and enjoyable one.

Moreover, group fitness provides a unique platform for social interaction and the formation of new friendships. Common goals and shared struggles naturally bring people together, creating a sense of camaraderie and mutual support. For instance, programs like CrossFit have a notorious reputation for fostering strong community bonds; members often celebrate each other's successes, whether it's achieving a personal best or completing a challenging workout. These social interactions are not limited to the time spent in the gym; many fitness groups organize social events outside of regular workout sessions, further strengthening the bonds between members. This social connectivity is crucial, as it can significantly enhance your commitment to a fitness regimen and make the overall experience more fulfilling.

The inclusivity of a fitness community is another critical factor that can greatly enhance your experience. An inclusive fitness community welcomes individuals of all skill levels and backgrounds, providing a supportive environment where everyone feels valued and capable of achieving their fitness goals. Creating such a community requires conscious effort and sensitivity from both instructors and participants. For example, fitness instructors can design programs that are adaptable to different fitness levels, ensuring that each participant can challenge themselves without feeling left behind. Participants, on the other hand, can foster an inclusive atmosphere by encouraging one another and respecting each individual's unique journey and pace.

A psychologically safe environment within fitness groups is essential for fostering a sense of security and belonging among members. Psychological safety means that members feel confident that they will not be exposed to discrimination, criticism, or any form of negative judgment based on their abilities or personal characteristics. This safety is crucial for allowing individuals to express themselves and engage fully without fear of embarrassment or rejection. For instance, a running club that celebrates each member's progress, regardless of pace, promotes a sense of achievement and belonging. Ensuring such an environment can encourage consistent participation and help individuals feel more connected to the group, enhancing both their physical and emotional well-being.

In essence, group fitness goes beyond physical health; it is a gateway to building stronger social connections and enhancing emotional health through community and inclusivity. As you continue to engage in these communal activities, you may find the social benefits to be just as rewarding as the physical ones. Each class, session, or event becomes an opportunity not just to enhance your fitness but to deepen your social interactions, broaden your support network, and enrich your overall quality of life.

Online Communities for Holistic Health Support

In today's digital age, the internet has revolutionized the way we seek and share health information. For anyone embarking on a journey toward holistic health, online communities—from dedicated forums and social media groups to specialized health apps—offer a wealth of resources right at your fingertips. These platforms can connect you with like-minded individuals across the globe, providing a space to share experiences, advice, and support. Imagine logging onto a forum and finding a thread discussing natural remedies for anxiety, or joining a Facebook group where members share their favorite vegetarian recipes. These interactions not only enrich your knowledge but also provide emotional support, making your wellness journey less isolating.

However, while these communities offer numerous benefits, they also come with their own set of challenges. The accessibility and anonymity of the internet can sometimes lead to the spread of misinformation. It's crucial to approach the information shared in these spaces with a critical eye. Verify the credibility of the sources and cross-check facts with reputable health websites or professionals. Additionally, the anonymity that makes it easy to share sensitive health issues also opens the door to potential cyberbullying or negative interactions. It's important to navigate these communities with caution, protecting your mental well-being by not engaging in or escalating online conflicts.

To foster positive interactions within these virtual spaces, it's essential to practice respectful communication and protect your privacy. Engage constructively by sharing your experiences and knowledge without making generalizations or giving unsolicited advice. Be mindful of the personal information you share, and set strict privacy settings on your accounts to control who can see your posts. By cultivating a respectful and cautious approach, you can make the most out of online communities without compromising your safety or peace of mind.

These online platforms can also serve as a bridge to real-world interactions, enhancing the tangible community support system. Many online groups organize local meetups or health-related events, providing an opportunity to connect face-to-face with those you've interacted with virtually. Participating in these events can deepen your connections and provide a sense of community that extends beyond the digital realm. Moreover, you can leverage these networks to initiate or participate in local wellness projects—such as starting a community garden or organizing a health fair—that benefit not just individual members but also the broader community. By integrating online interactions with real-world activities, you can enrich your holistic health journey with both global insights and local engagements, creating a well-rounded approach to wellness that leverages the best of both worlds.

Wellness Workshops and Local Events

Stepping into a local wellness workshop or attending a vibrant health fair isn't just about learning new things. It's about immersing yourself in a community that shares your interest in living better, healthier lives. Imagine the synergy of a group fitness challenge or the interactive learning at a seminar where every attendee is eager to improve their health and well-being. These local events offer invaluable opportunities to connect, learn, and grow in ways that daily routines seldom allow. They serve as essential platforms for exchanging ideas, encouraging each other, and even finding new inspiration to take your wellness journey further.

When you participate in these local gatherings, the educational benefits are immense. Seminars can introduce you to the latest health trends and evidence-based practices that you might not encounter online or in books. Health fairs often bring together a variety of practitioners, from nutritionists and personal trainers to holistic health experts, providing a broad spectrum of insights and services under one roof. Here, you can ask direct questions and receive immediate feedback, helping you better understand and navigate your health choices. Moreover, the social opportunities at these events are just as beneficial. Connecting with people who are also on their wellness paths can lead to new friendships and provide a sense of community that supports your own health goals. These interactions often create a motivational atmosphere that can reignite your passion for health and inspire you to pursue new practices or revitalize your existing routines.

Organizing community wellness activities can be a fulfilling endeavor that not only benefits your health but also enriches your local area. If you're inspired to bring wellness closer to home, start by identifying the needs and interests of your community. Perhaps a survey or informal conversations at local gatherings could provide insights into what topics or activities would garner the most interest. Once you've pinpointed these interests, reaching out to local health professionals, fitness instructors, or nutrition experts—who might be willing to participate or speak at your event—can add substantial value. Securing a venue is next, whether it's a community center, a park, or a school gym, depending on the size and nature of the event. Promoting your event through local businesses, schools, and social media will help attract a wider audience. Remember, the key to a successful event lies in good planning, clear communication, and a dash of creativity to make the experience both informative and enjoyable for all participants.

Incorporating both traditional and modern health practices into your events can cater to diverse preferences and increase the educational value of your gatherings. For instance, combining yoga sessions with workshops on the latest fitness technologies can appeal to different age groups and interests, providing a comprehensive overview of health and wellness. This approach not only broadens the appeal of your event but also encourages attendees to explore various facets of health and wellness that they may not have considered before.

Reflecting on successful events can provide valuable lessons and inspiration. Take, for example, a community that organized a "Health and Harmony" fair, which combined local artisan foods, yoga classes, and seminars on mental health. The event was a hit, drawing a large crowd and sparking interest in monthly follow-up meetings. Such successes underscore the positive impact that well-planned wellness events can have on a community's health and cohesion. They not only provide immediate health benefits and learning but also foster a collaborative spirit that can lead to sustained health initiatives within the community.

As we wrap up this chapter on community building through wellness workshops and local events, remember that these activities are more than just educational opportunities—they are a catalyst for creating healthier, more connected communities. By participating in or organizing these events, you contribute to a collective effort to enhance well-being on both a personal and community level. This chapter has equipped you with the knowledge to engage more deeply in your community's health landscape, whether by attending events, sharing your knowledge, or taking the lead in organizing. Each step you take builds towards a healthier, more vibrant community, reflecting the true essence of holistic wellness that extends beyond individual pursuits and nourishes the entire community.

"Holistic wellness thrives on social wellness and community building, weaving a tapestry of interconnected lives that support and uplift each other."

Chapter 7 Wellness Plan: Social Wellness and Community Building

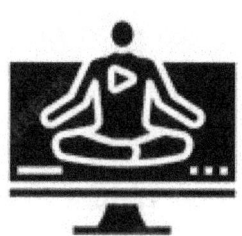

Activity: Cultivating Social Wellness

Take proactive steps to enhance your social wellness and build a supportive community around you. Reflect on each activity, document your experiences, and use music to enrich your journey.

Building Supportive Relationships:
◆ Identify three key people in your life who form your support system.
◆ Reach out to each person and express your appreciation.
◆ Plan a meaningful activity with one of them (e.g., a coffee date, a walk, or a shared hobby).
☆ *Reflection:*
☆ *How did expressing appreciation affect your relationship?*

- ☆ *What did you enjoy about the shared activity?*

Communicating Needs and Boundaries:

- ◈ Identify a situation where you need to set a boundary or express a need.
- ◈ Use "I" statements to communicate this clearly and assertively.
- ☆ **Reflection:**
- ☆ *How did the conversation go?*
- ☆ *What was the response, and how did you feel afterward?*

Volunteering:

- ◈ Choose a local organization or cause to volunteer with.
- ◈ Dedicate at least one hour to volunteer work this week.
- ☆ **Reflection:**
- ☆ *What activities did you engage in during your volunteering?*
- ☆ *How did volunteering make you feel emotionally and physically?*

Group Fitness Participation:

- ◈ Join a group fitness class or a sports league.
- ◈ Attend at least one session.
- ☆ **Reflection:**
- ☆ *Describe the atmosphere and energy of the group.*
- ☆ *How did participating in the group activity affect your motivation and enjoyment of exercise?*

Engaging with Online Communities:

◆ Join an online health or wellness community (e.g., forum, Facebook group, health app).

◆ Participate in a discussion or share an experience.

☆ *Reflection:*

☆ *What did you learn from the online community?*

☆ *How did it feel to connect with like-minded individuals?*

Attending Wellness Workshops or Events:

◆ Find a local wellness workshop or health event to attend.

◆ Participate actively and network with other attendees.

☆ *Reflection:*

☆ *What new information or skills did you learn?*

☆ *How did attending the event enhance your sense of community?*

Organizing a Community Wellness Activity:

◆ Plan and organize a small wellness activity (e.g., a group walk, a healthy potluck, or a meditation session).

◆ Invite friends, family, or community members to join.

☆ *Reflection:*

☆ *How did organizing and participating in the event feel?*

☆ *What was the feedback from the participants?*

Music Suggestions:

◈ Energetic Playlist:

☆ *Curate a playlist of uplifting and energizing songs for group activities and fitness classes. Include tracks that foster a sense of community and motivation.*

◈ Calming Tunes for Reflection:

☆ *Create a playlist of soothing and reflective instrumental music for journaling and relaxation. Use these tunes to create a peaceful environment for your reflective activities.*

Acknowledge Your Effort:

Take a moment to celebrate the efforts you've made to build and strengthen your social wellness. Reflect on the positive changes and connections you've experienced. Recognize that each step you take towards building supportive relationships and engaging with your community contributes to your holistic health and well-being.

Remember, social wellness is a continuous journey. Each interaction and activity enriches your life, helping you create a network of support and connection that uplifts and sustains you through life's challenges and joys. Keep nurturing these relationships and communities, and enjoy the profound benefits they bring to your overall well-being.

Chapter 8

Adapting Wellness Into Your Unique Lifestyle

Tailoring Wellness Practices for Different Life Stages

Navigating through life's stages can sometimes feel like trying to stitch a quilt from different fabrics, each piece representing a different phase with its unique texture and color. From the vibrant, fast-paced days of youth, through the transformative years of midlife, to the reflective season of seniority, each stage demands different wellness strategies. Understanding and adapting these strategies to align with your life phase not only enhances your well-being but also ensures that your wellness journey is rich, fulfilling, and, most importantly, effective.

Identifying Needs by Life Stage

The beauty of life lies in its dynamism and diversity—qualities that are mirrored in our evolving wellness needs. During the energetic years of youth and early adulthood, the focus often leans towards maintaining high energy levels and managing stress, particularly from career building and social dynamics. As you transition into midlife, the narrative shifts slightly towards maintaining optimum physical health, managing the stress that comes with life's peak responsibilities, and preparing for a healthy older age. This preparation might involve more focused preventive health measures such as regular screenings and adopting a heart-healthy diet. When you step into the golden years, the focus pivots towards preserving mobility, cognitive function, and social engagement. Each stage builds upon the previous, and understanding this progression can help you tailor your wellness practices to better meet your changing needs.

Youth and Wellness

For young adults, integrating wellness amidst the whirlwind of establishing careers and navigating social landscapes can be daunting. Energy management becomes crucial. Simple practices like maintaining a balanced diet rich in whole foods can provide sustained energy throughout the day. Incorporating physical activities that align with your interests—be it yoga, cycling, or team sports—can significantly boost your physical and mental health. However, mental wellness should not be overlooked. Techniques such as mindfulness meditation or journaling can be powerful tools for managing stress and anxiety, fostering a sense of inner peace that supports your overall well-being.

Midlife Wellness Strategies

As you move into midlife, maintaining your physical health becomes increasingly important. This stage often involves juggling multiple roles—professional, parent, spouse, caregiver—all of which can take a toll on your health if not managed well. Stress management is key. Regular physical activity, such as brisk walking or swimming, can help mitigate stress while also combating the metabolic slowdown associated with aging. Additionally, this is a critical time to invest in preventive health measures. Regular health screenings, such as blood pressure checks, cholesterol levels, and diabetes screenings, become vital. These proactive steps can help you catch potential health issues early, making them easier to manage or even reverse.

Senior Health Focus

In the later years of life, the emphasis shifts towards maintaining mobility, cognitive function, and social connections. Adapting exercises to accommodate any physical limitations is crucial. Low-impact activities like tai chi, water aerobics, or chair yoga can be beneficial. These activities not only help maintain muscle strength and flexibility but also enhance balance, reducing the risk of falls. Nutrition also plays a pivotal role; diets rich in omega-3 fatty acids, antioxidants, and soluble fibers can support cognitive function and overall health. Social engagement, often overlooked, is critical during this stage. Participating in community activities or volunteer work can provide both mental stimulation and a sense of purpose, enriching your later years with joy and connectivity.

Adapting your wellness routine to suit your current life stage is not just about adding or modifying activities; it's about creating a harmonious blend of practices that resonate with your body's needs and your life's demands. This personalized approach ensures that your wellness journey is not only about longevity but about enhancing the quality of life at every stage. As you transition through life's different seasons, keep in mind that each stage offers unique opportunities for growth and health, and with the right strategies, you can thrive through them all.

Overcoming the Guilt of Self-Care

In today's fast-paced society, taking a moment for oneself can sometimes feel like a luxury or, worse, a mark of selfishness. This is especially true for those who juggle multiple roles—parents, caregivers, professionals—who often find themselves postponing their own needs to cater to others'. The stigma associated with self-care is rooted deeply in cultural narratives that praise tirelessness and criticize self-focus. However, dismantling these perceptions is crucial, not only for your well-being but also for maintaining your ability to care for others effectively.

Addressing the stigma involves reshaping how we perceive self-care, starting with recognizing that it is an absolute necessity, not a luxury. Psychological insights tell us that neglecting self-care can lead to burnout—a state of emotional, physical, and mental exhaustion caused by prolonged stress. This not only diminishes your ability to perform daily tasks but also affects your health and relationships negatively. It's essential to challenge the old paradigms that associate self-care with guilt. Instead, view it as a preventive strategy that keeps you healthy and energized, thus enabling you to be more present and supportive in the lives of those you care about.

Balancing self-care with responsibilities may seem like a daunting task, but it can be managed with the right strategies. Effective time management is key. Start by assessing how you currently spend your time. Identify activities that do not add value or joy to your life. Could these be minimized or eliminated? Next, prioritize tasks using the Eisenhower Box technique, which helps you decide on and prioritize tasks by urgency and importance, focusing on what truly needs your attention. Additionally, setting clear boundaries is crucial; it's okay to say no or delegate tasks to ensure you're not over-committing yourself. This not only helps prevent burnout but also frees up time to engage in rejuvenating activities that enhance your well-being.

Reinforcing the idea that self-care is a necessity involves a shift in mindset and culture within families, workplaces, and communities. It's about understanding that taking care of your health—physical, mental, and emotional—is fundamental to living a full and capable life. Research consistently shows that well-rested, mentally healthy individuals perform better at work and maintain healthier relationships. Encouraging a culture where taking time for mental health is normalized can lead to more productive and happy individuals. For instance, companies that implement policies supporting mental health days and encourage regular breaks see improved employee satisfaction and productivity.

To illustrate the positive effects of self-care, let's look at Maria, a healthcare professional and mother. Initially overwhelmed by her responsibilities, Maria attended a work-life balance workshop and learned to set firm boundaries and allocate time for hobbies. This not only boosted her mental health but also enhanced her engagement and productivity both at home and at work. Similarly, John, a senior software developer, incorporated short mindfulness walks into his workday, experiencing increased focus and reduced stress. These instances demonstrate how integrating self-care strategies can significantly improve personal and professional well-being, emphasizing its importance and effectiveness.

Integrating Wellness into the Workday

When you think about your workday, it's often a balancing act between productivity and well-being. But what if you could integrate both seamlessly? Workplace wellness programs are more than just a corporate trend; they are a pivot toward a healthier, more engaged workforce. Participating in or even initiating these programs can transform your work environment into a space that supports holistic health, encompassing exercise, mindfulness, and healthy eating initiatives. Imagine the boost in morale and reduction in stress when employees have access to structured wellness activities right at their workplace. These programs could range from organized group workouts to scheduled mindfulness sessions, all designed to reduce stress and promote health without stepping out of the office.

Now, let's talk about incorporating these wellness practices directly into your daily routine. Desk exercises and proper ergonomics play a crucial role here. It's easy to underestimate the strain that prolonged sitting can have on your body. Integrating simple exercises into your workday can significantly alleviate this. For instance, every couple of hours, you could perform stretches specifically designed for office environments—like neck rolls and wrist stretches—or even maintain a mini stepper under your desk for a quick cardio session. Pairing these physical activities with an ergonomic workstation setup—ensuring that your monitor is at eye level and your chair supports your lower back—can drastically reduce the risk of strain and injury, promoting better physical health and greater comfort throughout your workday.

Mental resets are equally important. They help maintain focus and reduce stress, key components in enhancing work performance and overall well-being. Simple practices like taking short meditative breaks or engaging in walking meetings can provide these mental refreshes. Imagine replacing a traditional conference room meeting with a walking meeting outside. This not only fosters a dynamic discussion but also incorporates physical activity into your agenda, hitting two birds with one stone. Additionally, mindfulness sessions, even if brief, can be incorporated throughout the day to help clear the mind and relieve stress. Techniques such as focused breathing or visualization can be done right at your desk and are effective methods for recalibrating your mental state, keeping you sharp and centered.

Balancing work and personal life is paramount, and it often starts in the workplace. Setting clear boundaries is essential; it's important to communicate effectively with your team about your availability and work hours to ensure you have time to recharge after work. Effective stress management also plays a crucial role. This could involve setting realistic daily goals, which helps in managing expectations and reducing the urge to overextend yourself. Furthermore, encouraging a culture that prioritizes wellness can lead to more sustainable work practices, including recognizing the signs of burnout and encouraging regular breaks among team members. These strategies not only enhance individual well-being but also foster a supportive and productive work environment.

Incorporating these elements into your workday isn't just about personal health; it's about fostering a workplace culture that values and actively promotes wellness. By integrating physical exercises, ergonomic solutions, mental health practices, and a well-balanced approach to work and life, you can create a more productive, enjoyable, and healthy work environment. This holistic approach not only benefits individual employees but also contributes to a more vibrant, energetic, and healthy workplace culture.

The Role of Personal Development in Wellness

Exploring the realms of personal development is akin to planting a garden of diverse experiences—it nurtures your mind, enriches your emotions, and cultivates a healthier, more resilient you. From learning a new language to picking up a musical instrument, or diving into a creative hobby like painting, each new skill or hobby you acquire doesn't just fill your time—it enhances your cognitive abilities, boosts your emotional well-being, and integrates seamlessly with your holistic health goals. This fusion of lifelong learning and wellness is not just about adding activities to your busy schedule; it's about enriching your life's tapestry with vibrant threads of growth and satisfaction.

Lifelong Learning and Wellness

The connection between personal development and wellness is profound. Engaging in continuous learning has been shown to improve brain function, enhance emotional regulation, and increase life satisfaction. When you challenge your brain with new skills, you're essentially strength-training it, making it stronger and more adaptable. This mental agility can translate into better problem-solving skills, a sharper memory, and delayed cognitive decline as you age. Moreover, the joy and satisfaction derived from mastering a new skill can be a significant mood booster, reducing stress and contributing to your overall happiness.

Personal development also fosters a sense of accomplishment and self-efficacy. When you learn to play a new instrument, for instance, not only do you enjoy the music you create, but you also build confidence in your ability to tackle new challenges. This confidence can permeate other areas of your life, improving your overall approach to challenges and setbacks. Additionally, hobbies and continuous learning often provide opportunities for social interaction, whether through classes, clubs, or online communities. These social connections are vital for emotional health, offering support, inspiration, and camaraderie.

Setting Personal Growth Goals

When integrating personal development into your wellness strategy, setting clear, achievable goals is crucial. These goals should be specific, measurable, achievable, relevant, and time-bound (SMART). For instance, if you're interested in photography, a SMART goal could be, "Enroll in an introductory photography course at the community center and complete it by the end of the quarter." This goal is specific (take a course), measurable (complete the course), achievable (introductory level), relevant (interest in photography), and time-bound (by the end of the quarter).

Setting personal growth goals helps maintain your focus and makes the process of learning new skills more structured and rewarding. It also allows you to track your progress, which can be incredibly motivating. Reflect on your interests and how they align with your long-term wellness goals. For example, if stress reduction is a priority, you might choose activities known for their calming effects, like yoga or knitting. Alternatively, if enhancing cognitive function is your goal, learning a new language or instrument can be particularly beneficial.

Integrating Personal and Professional Growth

Balancing personal interests with professional development can enhance both your career and personal life. For many, professional growth is closely linked to personal satisfaction. However, it's important to find harmony between the two, ensuring that one does not overshadow the other. For instance, if you're a marketing professional interested in graphic design, taking a course in this field can enrich your skill set, making your work more fulfilling and opening up new career opportunities. Similarly, developing skills like public speaking or project management can boost your confidence and performance in personal endeavors like community volunteering or running a club.

Integrating personal and professional development involves continuous reflection and adjustment. It's about understanding how the skills you acquire in one area can benefit the other. This holistic approach not only leads to a more satisfying career but also enriches your personal life, making you a more well-rounded, content, and capable individual.

Resources for Personal Development

Fortunately, the resources available for personal development are vast and varied. Books, online courses, workshops, and podcasts can provide the guidance and inspiration you need to embark on your learning journey. Websites like Coursera or Udemy offer a plethora of courses in virtually any field imaginable, from science and technology to art and music. Local community centers, libraries, and colleges frequently provide classes and workshops that can offer both learning opportunities and a chance to connect with like-minded individuals.

Choosing resources that fit your learning style, schedule, and budget is key. For those with tight schedules, podcasts or audiobooks can be a perfect fit, offering the flexibility to learn while commuting or during other routine activities. For hands-on learners, workshops or physical classes provide immediate feedback and engagement that can be crucial for mastering new skills. Whatever resources you choose, ensure they align with your goals and provide the level of depth and engagement you need to stay motivated and inspired on your path to personal and professional fulfillment.

By weaving personal development into the fabric of your wellness strategy, you're not just learning new things; you're enhancing your overall quality of life, and building a resilient, capable, and satisfied self. Whether through developing new skills, setting growth-oriented goals, balancing personal and professional development, or utilizing diverse resources, the journey of personal development is a fulfilling path that promotes a healthier, happier you.

Keeping Wellness Engaging and New

Maintaining an engaging and fresh approach to your wellness routine is much like keeping a garden; it requires variety, attention to seasonal shifts, and the integration of new tools and technologies to thrive. Let's explore how you can invigorate your fitness and nutrition regimen, weave social wellness activities into your routine, adapt your practices to align with the changing seasons and harness innovative wellness technologies to keep your wellness journey lively and enjoyable.

Variety in Fitness and Nutrition

Sticking to the same workout routine or meal plan can quickly become tedious, leading to a plateau not just in your physical progress but in your enthusiasm as well. Injecting variety into your fitness and nutrition regimen can rekindle your interest and boost your motivation. Consider incorporating new forms of exercise into your routine. If you've always been a runner, why not try a dance class or take up swimming? Each sport engages different muscle groups and can be refreshing mentally and physically. Similarly, exploring new dietary changes can revitalize your interest in healthy eating. Enroll in a cooking class to master a cuisine you're unfamiliar with, or challenge yourself to a 'vegetable of the week' club where you try new or unusual vegetables in your meals. These changes keep your diet exciting and can lead to new discoveries about foods and cooking techniques that benefit your health.

Social Wellness Activities

Incorporating a social element into your wellness practices can dramatically enhance your engagement and commitment. Humans are inherently social beings, and we thrive on connection. Participating in group activities, whether joining a hiking club, enrolling in a group meditation class, or attending a fitness boot camp, provides not only companionship but also the motivation for shared goals. These activities allow you to connect with others who are on similar wellness paths, offering mutual encouragement and making the activities more enjoyable. The camaraderie developed in these social settings can be a powerful motivator, turning the solitary pursuit of wellness into a shared endeavor that brings joy and enhanced commitment to your health goals.

Seasonal Wellness Changes

Just as nature cycles through seasons, your wellness routine can benefit from adjustments that align with seasonal changes. This keeps your routine aligned with the natural world and prevents monotony from creeping into your activities. During the warmer months, take advantage of the weather to engage in outdoor activities such as cycling, outdoor yoga, or beach volleyball. As the weather cools, transition to indoor activities like joining a gym, trying indoor rock climbing, or swimming in an indoor pool. Seasonal changes can also be reflected in your diet; summer might focus on salads and smoothies while winter shifts to warm soups and roasted vegetables. Embracing the rhythm of the seasons keeps your activities fresh and attuned to the natural environment, enhancing your physical and mental well-being.

Innovative Wellness Tools and Tech

The ever-evolving landscape of technology offers new avenues to enhance your wellness practices. From fitness trackers that monitor your physical activity and sleep patterns to apps that provide guided meditation sessions, technology can be a valuable ally in your wellness journey. Wearable devices can help you stay on track with your fitness goals by providing real-time data on your performance and progress. Similarly, virtual reality experiences can offer immersive meditation or yoga sessions that transport you to calming environments, enhancing your relaxation and mindfulness practices. Apps that track your dietary intake and offer nutritious recipes can make maintaining a healthy diet easier and more enjoyable. By integrating these technological tools into your wellness regimen, you can add an element of fun and discovery, keeping your routine engaging and tailored to your evolving needs.

As you continue to explore these strategies, remember that the key to a vibrant wellness journey lies in staying curious and open to new experiences. Whether through trying new physical activities, connecting with others, adapting to the seasons, or integrating cutting-edge technology, there are endless opportunities to infuse excitement and novelty into your path to health and well-being. Keep exploring, keep experimenting, and keep enjoying every step of your wellness adventure.

Reviewing and Renewing Your Wellness Goals Annually

Reflecting on your wellness journey once a year isn't just about checking boxes; it's a crucial practice that helps align your actions with your evolving life circumstances and personal aspirations. It's like pausing on a hike to ensure you're still on the right path and making adjustments to reach the summit efficiently. This annual review is your opportunity to look back on what you've achieved, learn from what didn't go as planned, and set new goals that ignite your motivation. It's about maintaining a dynamic approach to your wellness, ensuring that your strategies remain relevant and motivating as your life changes.

Importance of Regular Reviews

Conducting regular reviews of your wellness goals serves multiple purposes. It allows you to see the progress you've made, which can be incredibly motivating. Reflecting on the successes, even the small ones, can fuel your desire to continue. More importantly, this review process helps you identify strategies that may no longer be effective or relevant. Life changes—perhaps you've moved to a new city, changed jobs, or experienced significant changes in your personal life—these shifts can all impact your wellness routine. By taking the time to assess your goals annually, you can make informed decisions about what to continue, what to stop, and what new goals you might want to pursue. This adaptability is key to maintaining a wellness routine that fits your current lifestyle and continues to bring you joy and health.

Setting SMART Goals

To ensure your wellness goals are clear and reachable, each one should be SMART—Specific, Measurable, Achievable, Relevant, and Time-bound. This framework not only guides your planning process but also enhances the likelihood of achieving your goals. For instance, instead of setting a vague goal like "get fit," a SMART goal would be "attend three yoga classes per week for the next three months." This goal is specific (attend yoga classes), measurable (three times a week), achievable (a realistic number of classes per week), relevant (contributes to your fitness), and time-bound (for the next three months). Using this structured approach in your annual planning helps turn abstract aspirations into actionable steps, making it easier to track progress and make adjustments as needed.

Celebrating Achievements and Learning from Setbacks

Each review is a chance to celebrate your successes and learn from the setbacks. When assessing your past year, take note of the achievements, no matter how small. Did you stick to your goal of meditating each morning? Did you make dietary changes that improved your health? Celebrating these victories reinforces your efforts and boosts your confidence. Likewise, it's important to reflect on the goals you didn't meet. Understanding why certain goals were not achieved can provide valuable insights. Was the goal too ambitious? Did unforeseen circumstances interfere? Analyzing these setbacks helps you learn and grow, ensuring that your future goals are more aligned with your capabilities and life situation.

Planning for Upcoming Years

Looking forward involves anticipating changes in your life that might impact your wellness routine. Maybe you're approaching a significant birthday, anticipating career changes, or your children are growing older, and your daily schedule will be different. These life events can significantly impact your wellness needs and the time you have available for wellness activities. By planning with these changes in mind, you can adapt your goals so that they continue to be relevant and achievable. For example, if you know a busy work period is approaching, you might focus on stress management techniques rather than intensive physical fitness goals. Planning for the future with foresight allows you to maintain continuity in your wellness journey, adapting smoothly to life's ebbs and flows.

As you wrap up your annual wellness review, take a moment to appreciate the journey you've been on. The insights you gain from this reflective process are invaluable, helping you to sculpt a wellness plan that not only meets your needs but also sparks joy and fulfillment in your everyday life. Looking ahead, you're equipped not just with goals, but with a deeper understanding of how to live well, no matter what life throws your way. Moving forward, you'll continue to refine, adjust, and thrive, carrying with you the lessons learned and the successes celebrated.

<u>Next Steps</u>

As we close this chapter on reviewing and renewing your wellness goals, remember that this process is an integral part of living a mindful, healthy life. It's about taking control of your well-being, celebrating your progress, and learning from every experience. Up next, we'll explore how to integrate these principles into broader aspects of your life, ensuring that wellness remains a joyful and rewarding part of your everyday existence.

> *"Embracing wellness within your unique lifestyle transforms health into a personal journey, harmonizing your well-being with your individual needs and aspirations."*

Chapter 8 Wellness Plan: Adapting Wellness Into Your Unique Lifestyle

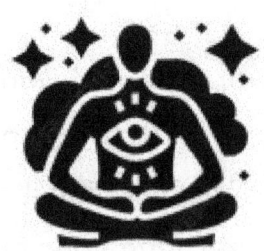

Activity: Annual Wellness Goals Review

Objective: Reflect on your past year's wellness journey, celebrate achievements, learn from setbacks, and set new goals for the upcoming year.

Step 1: Reflect on Achievements

★ List 3 wellness goals you achieved this year. Describe how you feel about these achievements.

Music Suggestion: "Happy" by Pharrell Williams

Step 2: Learn from Setbacks

★ Identify 2 wellness goals you didn't achieve. Reflect on the reasons why and what you learned from these experiences.

Music Suggestion: "Fix You" by Coldplay

Step 3: Set New SMART Goals

★ Write down 3 new wellness goals for the upcoming year. Ensure they are Specific, Measurable, Achievable, Relevant, and Time-bound (SMART).

Music Suggestion: "Eye of the Tiger" by Survivor

Step 4: Plan for Future Changes

★ Note any anticipated changes in your life (e.g., job change, moving) and how they might impact your wellness routine. Plan adjustments accordingly.

Music Suggestion: "Here Comes the Sun" by The Beatles

Step 5: Celebrate and Motivate

★ Write a short paragraph on how you will celebrate your achievements and stay motivated throughout the next year.

Music Suggestion: "Don't Stop Believin'" by Journey

End with Reflection

★ Spend 5 minutes reflecting on your wellness journey while listening to "What a Wonderful World" by Louis Armstrong.

Worksheet Summary:

- **Reflect on Achievements:** Celebrate your successes.

- **Learn from Setbacks:** Understand and grow from

what didn't work.

- **Set New SMART Goals:** Define clear, actionable goals.

- **Plan for Changes:** Prepare for future life events.

- **Celebrate and Motivate:** Keep your journey joyful and inspiring.

Chapter 9

Bonus Chapter: Ask the Wellness Coach

Real Questions. Practical Answers. No Judgment.

You asked, we answered. Here are some of the most common wellness questions I've received—from people just like you who are trying to live better without the overwhelm. Let's bust some myths, keep it real, and help you move forward with confidence.

Q: "Do I have to be vegetarian or vegan to be healthy?"

A: Not at all! While plant-based diets have great benefits, holistic wellness is about balance, not labels. You can be an omnivore and still make mindful choices—like eating more whole foods, cutting down on processed stuff, and being intentional with what goes on your plate.

Q: "I'm so busy. How do I even start a wellness plan?"

A: Start *tiny*. One glass of water when you wake up. Five minutes of deep breathing. A walk during your lunch break. You don't need an hour-long morning routine to feel better—you just need *consistency*, not perfection. Stack simple habits and build from there.

Q: "What's the best time of day to meditate or exercise?"

A: The best time is when *you'll actually do it*. Morning routines get a lot of hype, but if you're not a morning person, it's okay. Wellness isn't a race—it's a rhythm. Whether it's sunrise stretches or midnight journaling, the "right" time is the time that fits *your* life.

Q: "Is it okay to skip a day or fall off track?"

A: 100% yes. Life isn't a straight line, and your wellness journey won't be either. Progress isn't ruined by one skipped workout or a weekend of takeout. What matters is that you get back on track with *compassion*, not guilt. You're human. You're allowed to be flexible.

Q: "How do I deal with negative self-talk?"

A: Name it. Call it out. Replace it. Try saying:
- "This is a tough moment, but I'm doing my best."
- "I choose progress, not perfection."
- "I'm worthy of feeling well."

Your mind believes what you repeat. Choose to be kind to yourself.

Q: "Is holistic wellness expensive?"

A: It doesn't have to be! Many wellness practices are *free*: walking, breathing, journaling, sleeping better, drinking water. Sure, there are fancy products out there, but the foundation of true wellness is simple, sustainable, and accessible to all.

Q: "Where do I go from here?"

A: Use this book as your starting point. Revisit the parts that resonated. Pick *one* area—like nutrition, movement, or mindset—and take a small, doable step today. Wellness isn't a destination—it's a plan you can live with, one intentional choice at a time.

Q: "I want to eat healthy, but I hate cooking. Help?"

A: You don't have to be a chef to eat well. Think lazy-gourmet: rotisserie chicken + salad kit, smoothie packs, pre-chopped veggies. Batch cooking on Sundays can be a game-changer. Or go for no-cook options—Greek yogurt, nuts, fruit, overnight oats. Eating healthy doesn't have to mean hours in the kitchen.

Q: "What if my family isn't on board with my wellness goals?"

A: Focus on your lane. Be the inspiration, not the enforcer. Invite them in with curiosity: "Want to try this smoothie?" or "Join me for a walk?" Lead by example. Even small shifts in your energy can influence those around you more than lectures ever will.

Q: "How do I stay consistent when I keep losing motivation?"

A: Motivation is fickle. Build systems instead. Put your yoga mat where you can see it. Schedule walks like meetings. Use apps, reminders, playlists—whatever works. When motivation fades (and it will), your habits will carry you forward.

Q: "What's something I can do right now to feel better instantly?"

A: Breathe. Inhale for 4, hold for 4, exhale for 6. Do it 3 times. You've just calmed your nervous system. Then, get up and stretch, drink some water, or step outside. Tiny shifts = big impact when done consistently.

Q: "Can I include wine or dessert in a holistic lifestyle?"

A: Absolutely. Deprivation isn't wellness—*balance* is. Enjoy your glass of wine or a slice of cake mindfully and without guilt. The key is presence. Savor the moment, and let joy be part of your plan.

Q: "How do I know if I'm making progress?"

A: Progress isn't just weight or numbers. Ask yourself:
- Am I sleeping better?
- Do I feel calmer or more energized?
- Am I making better choices more often than not? Progress is personal. Celebrate the wins that don't show up on the scale.

Q: "What if I don't like gyms or traditional workouts?"

A: Great! Movement comes in many forms: dancing in your room, walking your dog, yoga on YouTube, biking, gardening, swimming, even cleaning with music on full blast. The best workout is the one you'll *actually enjoy*.

Q: "How do I unplug when I feel addicted to my phone?"

A: Try a mini digital detox:
- No screens during meals.
- Phone-free mornings for 30 minutes.
- Use "Do Not Disturb" mode after a certain time. Replace scrolling with something soothing—reading, journaling, stretching, or just sitting with a cup of tea.

Q: "Is holistic wellness spiritual or religious?"

A: It can be—but it doesn't have to be. Some find spiritual growth through prayer or meditation, others through nature, creativity, or service. Holistic wellness simply means you honor your whole self—body, mind, and spirit—whatever that means *to you*.

Q: "What if I mess up... again?"

A: You're not starting over. You're *starting from experience.* Wellness isn't about flawless execution. It's about showing up for yourself with grace, again and again. Forgive yourself. Then take the next best step.

Chapter 10

Conclusion

As we draw the curtains on this enriching journey through the realms of holistic wellness, let's take a moment to reflect on the path we've traveled together. From exploring the foundational aspects of holistic health to diving into practical nutrition, engaging in physical fitness, nurturing our mental and emotional well-being, and expanding into the spiritual and environmental dimensions of health, we've covered a vast landscape of knowledge and practices. Each chapter was designed not just to inform but to transform—encouraging you to weave these insights into the fabric of your daily life.

One of the most profound lessons we've embraced is the deep interconnectedness of our wellness dimensions. Your physical health influences your mental state, your emotional balance feeds into your spiritual well-being, and your environment impacts them all. This intricate web of connections underscores why a holistic approach is not just beneficial but essential for anyone seeking a truly balanced and healthy life.

Yet, as we've discovered, there is no universal blueprint for achieving wellness. Each of you brings your unique set of circumstances, needs, and preferences to the table. This diversity is not a challenge but a beautiful opportunity to tailor the principles we've discussed to craft a personal wellness journey that resonates deeply with your individual lifestyle and goals.

Embracing the spirit of continuous learning and adaptation is crucial as you forge ahead. The landscape of health and wellness is ever-evolving, with new insights, techniques, and technologies emerging regularly. Stay curious, remain flexible, and be willing to adjust your strategies as you grow and as new information becomes available. This openness will not only enhance your journey but also ensure it remains vibrant and fulfilling.

Now, I urge you to take that first, brave step toward integrating these holistic practices into your daily routine. Whether it's setting aside a few minutes each day for mindfulness, experimenting with nutritious recipes, or connecting with nature, each small step is a leap towards a fuller, more vibrant life.

Share your journey with others. There is immense power in community and shared experiences. By connecting with others who are also walking this path, you'll find not just companionship but also mutual inspiration and support. Together, you can celebrate successes, navigate challenges, and perhaps even inspire others to join in this beautiful pursuit of wellness.

Remember, the ultimate goal of embracing holistic wellness is to enrich your life, not just to extend it. It's about growing, learning, and thriving, reaching towards your fullest potential in all aspects of life. As you reflect on your personal wellness goals, think about what truly matters to you. Set intentions that are not just achievable but also deeply fulfilling.

Thank you sincerely for joining me on this journey. Your commitment to exploring and adopting a holistic approach to wellness is not just a gift to yourself but to those around you, as you become a beacon of health, balance, and vitality. Here's to moving forward with grace, strength, and joy on your continuous path to wellness. May you find the balance you seek, and may your life be all the richer for it. Cheers to good health, profound growth, and a vibrant life ahead!

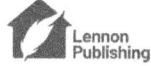

Thank You for Reading

We're so grateful you picked up *Holistic Living for Wellness*. We hope it brought you inspiration and practical tools for your wellness journey.

Enjoyed the book?

We'd love to hear your thoughts. Your review helps others discover the book and supports our growing wellness community.

Scan the QR code inside to leave a quick review, give us a like, or share your thoughts.

Every word you share means the world to us.

Thank you again for being part of this journey.

References

- AMA Journal of Ethics. (2008, March). Holistic medicine and Western medical tradition. https://journalofethics.ama-assn.org/article/holistic-medicine-and-western-medical-tradition/2008-03

- American Psychological Association. (n.d.). How stress affects your health. https://www.apa.org/topics/stress/health

- ATLWell. (n.d.). Gratitude journaling: A daily practice for mental health. https://www.atlwell.com/blog/gratitude-journaling

- Bija Bennet. (n.d.). 4 steps to creating a personal ritual. https://www.bijab.com/wellness-blog/how-to-create-a-personal-ritual/

- Cleveland Clinic. (n.d.). Music therapy: Types & benefits. https://my.clevelandclinic.org/health/treatments/8817-music-therapy

- Fitness Project. (n.d.). 8 quick and effective workouts for busy professionals. https://fitnessproject.us/blog/8-quick-and-effective-workouts-for-busy-professionals/

- Food Network. (n.d.). Water: How much should you drink every day? https://www.foodnetwork.com/recipes/photos/our-best-healthy-recipes-for-kids-and-families

- Global Wellness Summit. (n.d.). 12 wellness trends for 2023. https://www.globalwellnesssummit.com/press/press-releases/12-wellness-trends-for-2023/

- Greenleaf Communities. (n.d.). The many benefits of community gardens. https://www.greenleafcommunities.org/the-many-benefits-of-community-gardens/

- Harvard Health. (n.d.). Foods linked to better brainpower. https://thegirlonbloor.com/52-healthy-quick-easy-dinner-ideas-for-busy-weeknights/

- Healthline. (n.d.). 9 types of meditation: Which one is right for you? https://www.healthline.com/health/mental-health/types-of-meditation#:~:text=Not%20all%20meditation%20styles%20are,meditation%20author%20and%20holistic%20nutritionist.

- IHRSA. (n.d.). Creating an inclusive fitness club and sector. https://www.ihrsa.org/publications/creating-an-inclusive-fitness-club-and-sector-an-ihrsa-e-book/

- Mayo Clinic. (n.d.). Mindfulness exercises. https://www.mayoclinic.org/healthy-lifestyle/consumer-health/in-depth/mindfulness-exercises/art-20046356

- Mind. (n.d.). How nature benefits mental health. https://www.mind.org.uk/information-support/tips-for-everyday-living/nature-and-mental-health/how-nature-benefits-mental-health/

- Performance Health. (n.d.). 20 family fitness ideas beyond the gym. https://www.performancehealth.com/articles/20-family-fitness-ideas-beyond-the-gym/

- Psychological Healthcare. (n.d.). How life stages may affect your mental health. https://www.psychologicalhealthcare.com.au/blog/life-stages-mental-health/

- PubMed Central. (n.d.). Exploring the effects of volunteering on social, mental, and physical health. https://www.ncbi.nlm.nih.gov/pmc/articles/PMC10159229/

- PubMed Central. (n.d.). Foods that fight inflammation. https://www.ncbi.nlm.nih.gov/pmc/articles/PM

C4780815/

- PubMed Central. (n.d.). How the glycemic index can impact your mental health. https://www.ncbi.nlm.nih.gov/pmc/articles/PMC2805706/

- PubMed Central. (n.d.). Plant-based dietary patterns for human and planetary health. https://www.ncbi.nlm.nih.gov/pmc/articles/PMC9024616/

- PubMed Central. (n.d.). Sense of community and mental health: A cross-sectional analysis. https://www.ncbi.nlm.nih.gov/pmc/articles/PMC10314672/

- Self. (n.d.). 53 bodyweight exercises you can do at home. https://www.self.com/gallery/bodyweight-exercises-you-can-do-at-home

- Today. (n.d.). Walking benefits: The physical and mental benefits of walks. https://www.today.com/health/physical-mental-benefits-walking-t207904

- University of Georgia. (n.d.). 10 strategies for better time management. https://extension.uga.edu/publications/detail.html?number=C1042&title=time-management-10-strategies-for-better-time-management

- U.S. Department of Energy. (n.d.). Reducing electricity

use and costs. https://www.energy.gov/energysaver/reducing-electricity-use-and-costs

- Verywell Mind. (2024). 10 best mental health and therapy apps of 2024. https://www.verywellmind.com/best-mental-health-apps-4692902

- WebMD. (n.d.). What is holistic medicine and how does it work? https://www.webmd.com/balance/what-is-holistic-medicine

www.ingramcontent.com/pod-product-compliance
Lightning Source LLC
Chambersburg PA
CBHW020541030426
42337CB00013B/933